Breastfeeding

A Parent's Guide

TENTH EDITION

Amy Spangler, MN, RN, IBCLC

Contributors

Doraine Bailey, MA, *"Breastfeeding and Working"*
Rebecca F. Black, MS, RD/LD, IBCLC, *"Eating for Two"*
Karen Kerkhoff Gromada, MSN, RN, IBCLC, *"Breastfeeding More Than One Baby"*
Martha Hall, MSN, RN, IBCLC, and Sandra Jones, RD, MEd, IBCLC,
"Breastfeeding Beyond the First Year"
Elizabeth Hormann, EdM, IBCLC, *"Breastfeeding an Adopted or Previously Weaned Baby"*
Dennis L. Spangler, MD, *"Breastfeeding and Allergies"*
Mary Rose Tully, MPH, IBCLC, *"Breastfeeding a Premature Baby"*

Production

Design: Studio Rodrigo, *studiorodrigo.com,* New York, New York, USA
Editing and Production Management: Health Communication Connection, *healthcommunication.info*, Vienna, Virginia, USA
Illustrations: Mandy Root-Thompson, *meddrawstudio.com*, Westerville, Ohio, USA
Photography: Doug Jaeger, *dougjaeger.com,* New York, New York, USA; Gary Sloan Studios, *garysloan.com,* Northborough, Massachusetts, USA; Jensen Larson Photography, *jensenlarson.com,* Orlando, Florida, USA
Printing: Specialty Lithographing Co., *specialtylitho.com,* Cincinnati, Ohio, USA

Tenth Edition

21 22 23   1 2 3 4 5

ISBN 978-1-933634-43-2

To Den
for believing in me

Table of Contents

WHAT-IF'S

Author's Note

This book is designed so that each chapter provides complete information on the topic being discussed. As a result, some information appears in more than one chapter. The terms *milk* and *breast milk,* when used, refer to human milk.

WHY-TO'S

Chapter 1

Congratulations, You're About to Become a Parent!

You may think that once your baby is born the hard part is over. But the truth is the hard part is just beginning. A typical labor and birth can last up to 18 hours, but parenting lasts 18 years or more! Unfortunately, nothing can prepare you fully for the days and weeks to come. While reading books on baby care can be helpful, there is no substitute for on-the-job training. So take a deep breath and try to relax. You're about to become a parent.

Many parents are surprised to find that the excitement and anticipation they felt during pregnancy are quickly replaced by fear and frustration. With 8 hours of uninterrupted sleep a distant memory, even the most confident parents begin to doubt their ability to care for their baby.

I can do this.

Can I do this?

I can't do this!

I have to do this.

How can I do this?

Take a deep breath. Relax. Start slow. Focus your attention on learning how to feed, hold, and calm your baby. As your confidence in your ability to care for your baby grows, you will have more time for other tasks.

In some cultures, a new mother is expected to do everything by herself. Sound familiar? In other cultures, family members come and stay for weeks or even months to care for the mother while she cares for her baby. Wishful thinking? Either way, babies require a lot of work.

Don't expect everything to be perfect

Parents today are under a lot of pressure to do everything right. But when it comes to breastfeeding, there is no one size fits all approach. While some parents and babies—the lucky few—breastfeed with ease, most need to learn. So don't feel that you have to be an expert from the start. It may take several days or weeks before you and your baby know just what to do.

I thought breastfeeding was supposed to be natural.

I felt like a failure when I couldn't get my baby to latch on to my breast.

My baby slept all the time. I couldn't get him awake to breastfeed.

I was afraid to tell my friends that I had stopped breastfeeding.

If you are among the many mothers who have difficulty breastfeeding, you will find it reassuring to know that there is a solution to nearly every problem. Keep this book handy and refer to it as needed. Grandmothers, mothers, sisters, aunts, and friends may be eager to offer advice, but their knowledge of breastfeeding may be limited. So be sure to get help from a lactation professional who is trained to help breastfeeding mothers.

The more breast milk your baby receives, the greater the health benefits. Health professional organizations recommend exclusive breastfeeding for about the first 6 months and continued breastfeeding for at least 1–2 years. If you are unable to breastfeed exclusively, you and your baby will still benefit from whatever amount of breast milk you provide and from the closeness that comes with breastfeeding.

Some mothers, despite every effort, are unable to breastfeed. Fortunately, these situations are rare. If you happen to be a mother who can't breastfeed, it may help to know that infant formula can provide the calories and nutrients your baby needs to grow. And whether you breastfeed or not, the breast can still be a wonderful place to cuddle.

Expect the unexpected

No amount of planning can prepare you for the day when you are still in your nightgown at 3:00 in the afternoon, when your baby wants to breastfeed every hour, when a clean house and home-cooked meals are memories of a former life, and when sleep is more appealing than sex!

Parenting is the most important job you will ever hold, yet it is the job for which you will have the least amount of training. You will be on duty 24 hours a day, 7 days a week, 52 weeks a year—including weekends, nights, and holidays. There will be no benefits package—no pension plan, no paid vacation, no sick leave. There won't even be a salary. The only compensation you will receive will be a smile, a laugh, a hug, a first word, a first step, a first tooth. And looking back in years to come, without reservation or hesitation, you would do it all again!

Cherish every moment.

View this video to find out about the baby gooroo video series:

babygooroo.com/video/intro

Chapter 2

Benefits of Breastfeeding

Whether you plan to breastfeed or are unsure, knowing how breastfeeding benefits both you and your baby can be helpful.

Benefits to you

Health

- Women who breastfeed have less risk of prolonged or heavy vaginal bleeding after their babies are born.

- Breastfeeding helps the uterus return to its normal size.

- Breastfeeding reduces the risk of breast and ovarian cancer.

- Breastfeeding reduces the risk of postpartum depression.

Practical

- With breastfeeding there is no mixing, measuring, or clean-up, making nighttime feedings quick and easy.

- Breasts and babies are portable. Travel can be simple. With a little practice, mothers can breastfeed anywhere. Mothers who are shy or easily embarrassed might want to choose a quiet place where they will not be disturbed.

- Breast milk is always available and at just the right temperature! There is no need to worry about storage or refrigeration. This is especially important for mothers and babies in emergency situations where food supplies are limited or spoil easily.

Emotional

- Breastfeeding creates a special relationship between mother and baby, a closeness that comes with time and touch, a bond that lasts forever.

- Breastfeeding gives mothers a chance to rest during the day, something every new mother needs.

- With one hand free while breastfeeding, a mother can share her time and attention with other children or take care of personal needs.

Economic

- Parents who breastfeed save $1,500 or more in infant feeding costs during the first year.

- Breastfed babies experience fewer illnesses, doctor visits, and hospital stays. So parents who breastfeed save an average of $400 in health care costs during the first year.

- Breastfed babies are healthier, even if they are in child care. Parents who work outside the home miss fewer days of work and lose less income.

Environmental

- Breast milk saves energy. No gas, oil, coal, or electricity is needed to make breast milk. All you need is a breast, a baby, and a brain!

- Breastfeeding protects the environment. The only by-products are healthy mothers and babies!

- Breast milk comes conveniently packaged in individual servings. There is no need for glass or plastic containers.

Benefits to your baby

Health

Human milk...

- is the perfect food for your baby. It contains hundreds of nutrients plus special factors that protect your baby's health.

- changes to meet the needs of a growing baby, something formula cannot do.

- is easy to digest, so breastfed babies have less gas, colic, and spitting up.

Breastfed babies...

- have less diarrhea and constipation.

- are less likely to develop chronic bowel diseases such as ulcerative colitis, Crohn's disease, and celiac disease.

- have fewer respiratory infections and ear infections.

- are less likely to develop type 2 diabetes.

- are less likely to develop some childhood cancers such as leukemia and lymphoma.

- are less likely to become obese children.

Breastfeeding...

- promotes nervous system development and increases intelligence quotient (IQ).

- may reduce the risk of sudden infant death syndrome (SIDS), the leading cause of death in babies between 1 month and 1 year of age.

Emotional

- Breastfeeding gives babies a chance to touch, to smell, to hear, to see, to taste, to know their mothers from the first moment of birth.

Myths and misconceptions

Despite breastfeeding's many benefits, some women choose not to breastfeed or stop breastfeeding sooner than planned. Too often their decisions are based on misinformation. So whether you plan to breastfeed for 2 weeks, 2 months, or 2 years, knowing how to separate the myths from the facts will help you achieve your breastfeeding goals.

Will breastfeeding change the size and shape of my breasts?

Some women find that their breasts sag or droop after giving birth. This can happen whether you choose to breastfeed or decide to bottle-feed. These changes are due to heredity, age, and weight gain. The more weight you gain during pregnancy, the more your breasts will shrink or sag when the added pounds are lost.

Will breastfeeding be painful?

Breastfeeding can be painful at the start of a feeding when your baby first latches on to your breast. But as long as your baby is positioned correctly and has a good, deep latch, the pain should last only a few seconds.

Will breastfeeding tie me down?

During the early weeks, while you are building your milk supply and learning to breastfeed, frequent breastfeedings may limit your ability to come and go. But this gives you a chance to rest, to recover, and to get to know your baby. Once your milk supply is stable (about 6–12 weeks after birth), and your baby is breastfeeding less often, you will find it easier to come and go.

How can I keep my breasts from leaking?

Leaking often occurs in the early weeks when babies feed at irregular times. Fortunately leaking can be easily managed. See "Leaking," page 114. On a positive note, leaking is a good sign of milk production and milk release. Now only one task remains— getting the milk into your baby!

How can I tell if my baby is getting enough to eat?

You can be sure that your baby is getting enough to eat if she has frequent, runny, yellow stools (bowel movements) and is gaining weight. Fortunately, breastfed babies' stools have little or no odor!

Do I have to follow a special diet?

You will want to limit your intake of alcohol and caffeine. But you do not need to follow a special diet while breastfeeding, unless you find that certain foods make your baby fussy. See Chapter 10, "Eating for Two."

Do I need to stop breastfeeding if I get sick and need medicine?

Unless you have a serious illness like HIV/AIDS, the best protection for your baby is your milk, so keep breastfeeding. While most medicines are safe for breastfeeding mothers and babies, always check with your health care provider before you take any medicine, including medicine you buy over the counter (without a prescription). Remind your doctor that you are breastfeeding, so she can recommend medicine that is safe yet effective.

Can I breastfeed if I use marijuana?

Drugs used for recreation, as well as those prescribed by a health care provider to treat certain medical conditions, can pass into your milk and to your baby. While some drugs may be safe for breastfeeding babies, others are not. Unfortunately, we know very little about the effects of marijuana on breastfeeding babies. Some studies show that tetrahydrocannabinol (THC), the main active substance in marijuana, passes into human milk. But how much THC babies actually absorb and its effects are unclear. As marijuana becomes legal in more states within the United States, researchers hope to learn more about its short- and long-term effects. Until then, breastfeeding mom are urged to follow the American Academy of Pediatrics' recommendation and avoid marijuana use. Those moms who choose to use marijuana should talk with their baby's health care provider about the possible risks.

Will breastfeeding affect my sex life?

Some mothers have less desire for sex due to tiredness, fear of pregnancy, or fear of pain. Others find that breastfeeding alone provides enough touching and holding to satisfy their sexual needs. Still others are eager to resume having intercourse (sex). Discuss your feelings openly with your partner.

Many breastfeeding mothers have dryness in the vagina (birth canal) that can cause pain during intercourse. Putting a small amount of water-soluble lubricant, such as K-Y Jelly, around the opening of the vagina may be helpful.

When you have sex, you may have a climax or orgasm. An orgasm triggers the release of oxytocin from the brain. Oxytocin triggers the release of milk from the breasts. Some sexual partners feel like they have to come to bed thirsty or carry an umbrella! To limit the risk of leakage during sex, breastfeed your baby before making love.

If I breastfeed, can I still get pregnant?

Mothers who breastfeed exclusively or almost exclusively can delay pregnancy for about the first 6 months after birth. This method of natural child spacing is known as the lactational amenorrhea method (LAM). However, if your breastfeeding schedule or routine limits the frequency or length of breastfeedings or includes frequent use of breast milk substitutes, pregnancy is more likely to occur.

Ovulation (egg release) and menstruation (monthly bleeding) may not occur while you are breastfeeding, especially during the first 6–12 weeks. However, most women resume ovulation and menstruation while breastfeeding. Ovulation can occur before menstruation; therefore, do not assume that you are protected (safe) until after you have your first menstrual period.

If pregnancy is not desired, a safe method of birth control is suggested. Your choices include cervical cap, female condom, diaphragm, intrauterine device, tubal ligation, male condom, vasectomy, and spermicidal cream, foam, or jelly. Birth control pills that contain estrogen and progesterone (combination pills) are not recommended. However, birth control pills (minipills), implants (Implanon, Norplant), or injections (Depo-Provera) that contain only progesterone are thought to be safe. Your health care provider can help you decide which method of birth control is right for you.

If I get pregnant, can I still breastfeed?

Many mothers continue to breastfeed during pregnancy and have two different age babies or a baby and a young child at the breast after birth. This is called tandem nursing. Meeting the nutritional needs of three (mom, baby, and young child) can be challenging, so be sure to eat a variety of healthy, calorie-dense foods, drink to satisfy your thirst, and nap when your babies nap.

Your breast milk changes during pregnancy—a sign that your body is getting ready to feed a newborn. Milk volume decreases, sodium and protein increase, and lactose and glucose (sugars) decrease, causing your milk to look and taste more like colostrum. This change may cause your older child to lose interest in breastfeeding (child-led weaning), or breast tenderness, common during pregnancy, can make breastfeeding painful, and

you may decide it is time to wean (mother-led weaning). Weaning typically occurs when mom or baby decides the time is right.

Some mothers worry that breastfeeding will cause uterine contractions and increase the risk of premature labor. While there is no evidence to support this concern, if you have a history of premature labor, experience vaginal bleeding during pregnancy, or are pregnant with more than one baby, your doctor or midwife may suggest that you wean. See Chapter 12, "Weaning Your Baby."

More is better!

Any amount of breast milk is good for your baby. But research has shown that babies breastfed exclusively for 6 months are healthier—not just in infancy but for many years to come—compared to babies fed infant formula or a combination of formula and breast milk. Be patient. While breastfeeding may be challenging at first, the difficult parts are usually short-lived!

Moms and dads share their breastfeeding advice:

babygooroo.com/video/advice

How Breastfeeding Works

All you need is a breast, a baby, and a brain!

The human breast is an amazing organ that changes to meet the needs of your baby. You may find it easier to breastfeed if you know the parts of the breast and understand how each part works during lactation (milk production).

In order to breastfeed effectively, three things must take place: milk production, milk release, and milk transfer. For these three things to happen, you need a breast, a baby, and a brain.

Areola

Nipple

Montgomery's gland

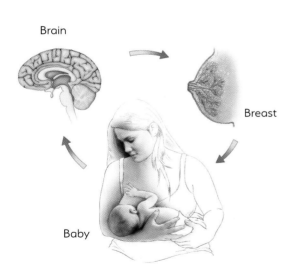

Brain

Breast

Baby

All you need to breastfeed is a breast, a baby, and a brain.

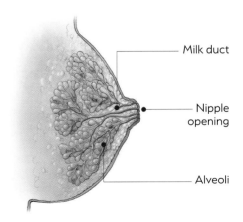

Milk duct

Nipple opening

Alveoli

The human breast has many parts, each with a special function.

When your baby begins to breastfeed, a message is sent to your brain. Your brain receives the message and sends a signal to the pituitary gland, a small group of cells attached to the base of the brain. The pituitary gland receives the signal and releases two hormones, prolactin and oxytocin. Prolactin tells your breast to make milk (milk production). Oxytocin tells your breast to release milk (milk release). Your baby then removes milk from your breast through breastfeeding (milk transfer). The more milk your baby takes, the more milk you make!

Oxytocin also causes uterine contractions which control uterine bleeding and help your uterus return to its nonpregnant size.

For more on milk production, milk release, and milk transfer, keep reading.

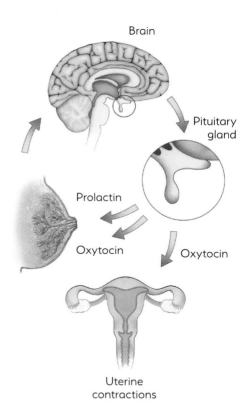

Infant suckling causes the release of prolactin and oxytocin from the pituitary gland.

Milk production

Breast milk is produced in the alveoli, grape-like sacs located inside the breast. There are two types of cells in the alveoli—secretory cells and myoepithelial cells. Secretory cells change fat and protein into milk. Myoepithelial cells contract and move milk from the alveoli into the milk ducts.

Milk production begins during pregnancy. But only a small amount of milk is produced, due to the presence of two hormones, progesterone and estrogen. These two hormones limit the release of prolactin, the milk-producing hormone. Progesterone and estrogen are made by the placenta, an organ that grows inside your uterus during pregnancy and nourishes your baby.

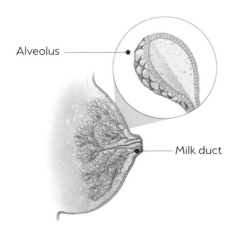

Alveolus

Milk duct

Milk production takes place in the alveoli, grape-like clusters of cells inside the breast.

After your baby is born, uterine contractions push out the placenta, causing progesterone and estrogen levels to fall. Prolactin levels then rise, triggering an increase in milk production. The increase in prolactin levels and milk production happens over a period of 3–5 days. However, if part of the placenta is left in the uterus after birth, prolactin levels stay low and milk production is delayed until the placenta is removed.

Breastfeeding should begin as soon as possible after birth—ideally within the first hour. The amount of milk you produce depends on the amount of milk your baby removes from your breasts. Early, frequent breastfeedings (at least eight feedings in each 24-hour period) will usually produce a good supply of milk. Prolactin levels increase two-fold each time your baby breastfeeds. This increase in prolactin has a relaxing effect on you and your baby—an added benefit of breastfeeding!

Milk release

When your baby begins to breastfeed, the following occur:

- Infant suckling signals the nerves inside the nipple to send a message to the brain—"Hungry baby!"

- The brain receives the message and signals the pituitary gland to release prolactin and oxytocin.

- Prolactin causes cells in the alveoli to make milk.

- Oxytocin causes cells around the alveoli to contract. These contractions move milk from the alveoli into the milk ducts.

- Oxytocin also causes milk to be released through the nipple openings.

This flow of milk through the breast is called the let-down reflex or milk-ejection reflex. It may take several seconds or several minutes for the release of milk to occur. It may also take several days or weeks for the let-down reflex to develop fully.

Factors that affect milk release include:

- embarrassment

- lack of confidence

- lack of encouragement and support

- pain

- stress

- tiredness

Milk transfer

Milk transfer is essential to effective breast-feeding. Some babies breastfeed often enough (eight or more times in each 24 hours) but they don't transfer (remove) milk from the breast.

Correct positioning of your baby *at* and *on* the breast is the key to milk transfer. When your baby is positioned correctly *at* the breast, his chin, chest, and knees face the breast. When your baby is positioned correctly *on* the breast, his mouth is opened wide—as if he is yawning—and is filled with breast.

Correct
positioning

Incorrect
positioning

Correct positioning of your baby *at* and *on*
your breast is the key to milk transfer.

Your baby forms a seal, using his lips and cheeks. This seal creates negative pressure, which helps to keep the nipple and the surrounding breast tissue in place.

When a let-down reflex occurs, newly produced milk flows through the milk ducts. Your baby lowers his tongue and increases the vacuum, allowing milk to flow into his mouth. The tongue is then raised. This reduces the vacuum, compresses the nipple, and triggers a swallow.

Hearing or seeing your baby swallow is one sign of milk transfer. You may also see milk leaking from one breast while your baby breastfeeds from the opposite breast.

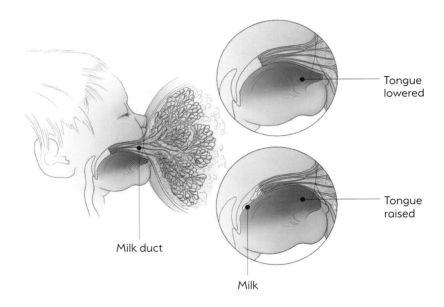

Tongue lowered

Tongue raised

Milk duct

Milk

When your baby is positioned correctly, your nipple is at the back of your baby's mouth and your milk ducts are compressed between the roof of your baby's mouth above and his tongue below.

Maintaining a milk supply

The signal for continued milk production is the removal of milk from the breast through breastfeeding (infant suckling) or breast expression (by hand or with a pump). Infant suckling causes a sudden increase in the level of prolactin. Prolactin plays an important role in maintaining milk production, but it does not affect milk volume. How much milk you make depends on the amount of milk your baby removes from your breasts. This is the process of supply and demand. The more milk your baby removes from your breasts, the more milk you will make.

When you delay or skip feedings and milk stays in your breasts, the milk causes an increase in pressure. This pressure slows the flow of blood to the alveoli and causes a decrease in milk production. As long as your baby continues to breastfeed, you will continue to make milk. However, if you limit the amount of breastfeeding by following a rigid feeding schedule or giving your baby water or formula supplements or a pacifier, your milk supply will decrease.

Human milk

Human milk goes by a variety of names (colostrum, transitional milk, and mature milk) depending on the stage of lactation. Although each contains similar nutrients, they vary in content and volume. From 0 to 5 days after birth, colostrum is produced; from 5 to 10 days, transitional milk is produced; and after 10 days, mature milk is produced. The shift from colostrum to mature milk is gradual and may occur unnoticed. The rate of change can vary depending on whether this is your first, second, or third baby and depending on how early and often your baby breastfeeds.

Colostrum

Colostrum is the first milk your breasts make. It can be thick and yellow or clear and runny. It is present during the last months of pregnancy and the first days after birth. Colostrum is high in protein, low in fat, and rich in antibodies that protect your baby from infection. Colostrum is often referred to as your baby's first immunization. It also acts as a natural laxative, causing your baby's bowels to move and reducing your baby's risk for jaundice. This explains why frequent feedings, starting within the first hour of birth, are important.

Transitional milk

Both the content and volume of transitional milk change gradually over a period of 5 to 10 days. The rate of change is often slower in first-time mothers. If you have had a prior pregnancy or have breastfed before, mature milk may appear sooner. During this period, the amount of sugar, fat, and calories increases, while the amount of protein and antibodies decreases, until the levels of mature milk are reached.

Mature milk

Mature milk was earlier thought to have two parts, foremilk and hindmilk. Foremilk was obtained at the start of a feeding and hindmilk at the end. And while it's true that milk obtained at the start of a feeding contains less fat than milk obtained at the end of a feeding, fat content varies widely, depending on the length of time between feedings.

To ensure that your baby gets the nutrients and calories she needs to grow, follow your baby's lead. Breastfeed at the first sign of hunger, and continue until your baby is full. As long as your baby is gaining weight and the distance around her head (circumference) and her length are increasing, you can be sure she is getting enough to eat.

Human milk, unlike formula, changes to meet the needs of your baby. In fact, the nutrients in human milk change from the beginning to the end of a feeding, from morning to night, from month to month, from mother to mother, and even from breast to breast! Although a mother's diet or health can affect the nutrients in her milk, mothers on restricted diets and those who are poorly nourished are still urged to breastfeed.

To ensure that your baby gets the nutrients and calories she needs to grow, breastfeed at the first sign of hunger, and continue until your baby is full.

Chapter 4

Getting Ready to Breastfeed

Get ready. Get set. Go!

The best time to learn all that you can about breastfeeding is before your baby is born. Planning ahead will help you reduce the risk of problems and find solutions quickly if problems do occur. The more knowledge you have about breastfeeding, the easier breastfeeding will be once your baby arrives.

Caring for your breasts

Montgomery's glands are small pimple-like bumps in the darker part of your breast around your nipple (see page 12). Montgomery's glands produce an oily material that keeps your nipples clean and moist. No special care is needed before (or after) your baby is born. Simply wash your breasts with mild soap and water when you shower or bathe, and avoid the use of creams, lotions, and oils.

Nipple exercises or other types of nipple preparation should be avoided. These include nipple rolling or pulling, rubbing your nipples with a towel or washcloth, hand expression, and breast pumping. Nipple preparation does not prevent the tenderness and pain that can occur when you first begin to breastfeed. The best way to prevent pain and avoid nipple damage is to position your baby correctly on your breast.

During pregnancy you may find that your breasts get fuller, your areolas darken, the Montgomery's glands enlarge, and a small amount of colostrum can leak from your nipples. Some women experience no breast changes but still produce an ample supply of milk. If your breasts show no signs of change during pregnancy, let your health care provider know. Together you can monitor your baby's weight to ensure that she is getting enough to eat.

Choosing breastfeeding supplies

Maternity shops, baby stores, and lactation centers offer a wide variety of breastfeeding supplies, including nursing bras, breast pads, nursing pillows, nursing clothes, and breast pumps. But all you truly need are three items—a baby, a breast, and a brain! So before you buy items advertised as "essential," be sure the added convenience justifies the cost. For example, stretchy cotton T-shirts or blouses that button up the front offer easy access to the breast and can be a lot less expensive, and a lot sexier, than nursing tops. One of the many benefits of breastfeeding is cost savings. So before you stock up on unnecessary supplies, consider the following.

Nursing bras

You do not need to wear a bra during pregnancy or while breastfeeding. If you prefer to wear a bra, nursing bras can be handy. A nursing bra has flaps that open over each breast, so that you can breastfeed without removing your bra. Mothers who experience leaking may prefer to wear a nursing bra to hold breast pads in place.

Nursing bras can be purchased at maternity stores or lactation centers. For a proper fit, wait until the last weeks of your pregnancy. You may find it helpful to talk with a professional who is skilled at bra fitting. Choose comfortable bras with cotton cups, adjustable straps, and simple flap fasteners. Avoid bras with underwires or bras that are too tight or bind, making it difficult to remove milk from all parts of the breast. If you prefer a bra with underwires, remove the bra for one or two feedings during the day and at night. Lightweight "sleeping bras" can be worn at night to hold breast pads in place should leaking occur.

Breast pads

Breast pads are used to protect clothes from leaking milk. Breast pads come in all shapes and sizes and are usually made from cotton or wool. Some pads are meant to be used only once, while others can be washed and used over and over again. Breast pads can be thick or thin. Thin pads can be less visible under clothing, but they may need to be changed more often. Remember to change pads frequently, and avoid pads with waterproof liners that trap wetness against the skin.

Nursing clothes

You do not need to wear special clothes to breastfeed your baby, but some mothers find nursing tops and nightgowns handy. Nursing clothes have openings over the breasts that are hidden in folds of fabric. The openings allow you to breastfeed your baby while keeping your clothes in place. Nursing clothes can make it easier to breastfeed discreetly in public, but the extra cloth can be bulky as well, so you may want to try different styles.

Breast and nipple size and shape

Many women worry that the size or shape of their breasts will affect their ability to produce milk. Breast size and shape are determined mainly by fat deposits. Although fat deposits protect the milk-producing cells in your breasts, they do not affect milk production.

The Pinch Test will help you see if your nipples are flat or inverted.

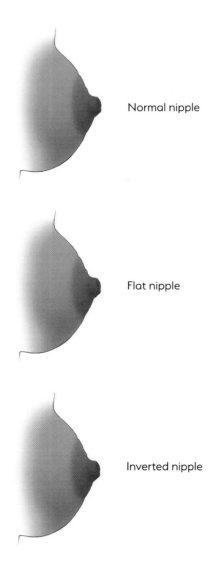

Normal nipple

Flat nipple

Inverted nipple

Nipples come in all shapes and sizes.

Nipple size and shape can make breastfeeding easier or harder for some babies. But most babies will learn to breast-feed on their mother's breasts if given the chance. All it takes is practice! The Pinch Test can help you decide if your nipples are normal, flat, or inverted.

- Place your thumb and first finger on your areola about 1 inch from your nipple.

- Press your thumb and finger together.

- A normal nipple will protrude or come out.

- A flat or inverted nipple will retract or sink in. (Truly inverted nipples are rare.)

If you are concerned about the size or shape of your nipples, talk with your health care provider early in your pregnancy.

If your nipples are truly flat or inverted and your baby has trouble breastfeeding, you may find a breast pump helpful. You can use the pump before each breastfeeding to gently pull your nipple out. See Chapter 7, "Your First Breastfeeding."

Breast shells

In the past, some women chose to wear breast shells during pregnancy to treat flat or invert-ed nipples. But researchers found that breast shells are seldom helpful and may actually do more harm than good. It is best to wait

A breast pump can be used before each breastfeeding to pull out flat or inverted nipples. (Examples shown, left to right, are made by Avent, Ameda, and Medela.)

until after your baby's birth to see if he has difficulty breastfeeding.

Nipple shields

A nipple shield is a device that can be used in special situations to aid attachment, support milk transfer, and assist breastfeeding. Babies who may benefit from the use of a nipple shield include premature babies who are unable to maintain a latch, babies who are accustomed to a bottle nipple and refuse to breastfeed, and babies of mothers with flat or inverted nipples. A nipple shield can be used

Nipple shields can make latch-on easier when a mother has a flat or inverted nipple. However, a nipple shield can limit milk production, milk release, and milk transfer.

at the start of a feeding to encourage your baby to latch on, and can then be removed after your baby begins to suckle and swallow. A nipple shield can also be used throughout the feeding.

Different types of nipple shields are available, and some are more effective than others. The thick rubber (latex) shields of the past are more likely to interfere with milk transfer compared to today's ultra-thin silicone shields. However, it's important to remember that all nipple shields are meant for short-term use until the breastfeeding problem is solved. Always check with your health care provider before using a nipple shield. If you decide to use a nipple shield, check your baby's weight often (at least weekly) so you can be sure that she is getting enough to eat.

Planning ahead

Caring for a new baby takes time, no matter how you choose to feed your baby. Try to complete as many tasks as possible before your baby is born.

• Prepare a space for your baby in your room.

• Get a crib or bassinet and a car seat that meet current safety standards.

• Take infant CPR, first aid, and baby care classes.

• Choose a health care provider for your baby.

• Make a list of nearby lactation support services.

• Prepare and freeze meals for later use.

• Write and send thank-you notes for baby gifts already received.

• Address and stamp envelopes if you plan to send birth announcements.

• Pay household bills early.

• Complete all work-related projects.

• Clean and organize your apartment or home.

• Last but not least, spend time with your partner. Once your baby arrives, time will be in short supply!

Moms share their thoughts on the hardest part of breastfeeding:
babygooroo.com/video/hardest

Learn more about the use of nipple shields:
babygooroo.com/handouts

Chapter 5

Especially
for Partners

Becoming a family

Families today come in all shapes and sizes—grandparents, fathers, mothers, brothers, sisters, boyfriends, girlfriends, and best friends. You can have a family of two, three, four, or more. No matter what type of family you have, the arrival of a new baby triggers a wide range of emotions. So take a deep breath, relax, and enjoy each moment, because it doesn't get any easier than this!

Breastfeeding benefits everyone who is an important part of your baby's life. A breastfed baby, warm and snug against your chest, gives you confidence in your ability to calm your baby.

Nighttime feedings are simple when there is no formula to mix, measure, or warm. In addition, breastfed babies are portable, good news for families on the go.

Learning to breastfeed

Learn all that you can about breastfeeding before your baby is born. While making milk is natural, breastfeeding is a skill that often requires practice. Sometimes a mother and baby know just what to do, but more often they need to learn.

This book will answer most of your questions, so be sure to read it carefully and keep it handy.

Watch as the nurses and lactation consultants assist your partner with breast-feeding, and ask them to show you how you can help.

Remember that babies (and mothers) need to breastfeed frequently and rest often, so you may need to limit the number of visitors and the length of visits. There will be plenty of time later for extended family and friends.

Accepting help with household chores

Accept all offers of help from people willing to cook, clean, do laundry, shop for food, or care for your partner. Refuse all offers of help from those who are interested only in caring for your baby.

In order to gain confidence in your ability to care for your baby, you and your partner need to practice your parenting skills.

Grandma already knows how to care for babies; now it is time for you and your partner to learn. But be sure to tell Grandma how much you appreciate her help as you learn to be a parent to her grandchild.

Getting to know your baby!

Breastfeeding is an important part of parenting, but equally important is the time you spend with your baby and the special moments you share. Find something you enjoy doing with your baby and make it a routine. Taking walks, splashing in the tub, listening to music, playing games, or simply watching TV or reading the newspaper are ways for you and your baby to spend time together and get to know one another.

Returning to "normal"

Many parents ask, "When will things get back to *normal?*" The truth is, never! Your idea of normal will need to change. You will need to adjust priorities and establish goals for a life that now includes another person. There may be little time at first for individual needs. However, as you learn to be a parent to your baby, remember to be a friend and lover to your partner.

Spend time getting to know your baby.

Despite all your efforts there will be good days and not so good days. Be prepared for the day when you arrive home to find your partner still in her nightgown. She and the baby are crying, the laundry needs to be done, and there is no dinner. Perhaps your day was just as bad! Instead of getting angry, put a load of clothes in the washing machine, take the baby for a walk (it will relax all of you), order food for dinner, and suggest that your partner make a cup of tea and take a warm bath. She will love you for understanding, and it will keep you both from saying things you might later regret.

Providing encouragement and support

In Chapter 2, "Benefits of Breastfeeding," you learned that breastfeeding is good for the entire family. (If you haven't read Chapter 2 yet, it's not too late!) Studies show that mothers are 10 times more likely to breastfeed if they have the support of their partner.

So why don't all partners encourage mothers to breastfeed? The fact is that most partners do support breastfeeding—at first. But early support is often short-lived.

Knowing how other parents feel might help you manage your feelings better.

I didn't realize how much I would miss the quiet nights and childless days.

Sometimes I'm angry at the baby for changing our lives.

Sometimes I'm angry at my partner for spending so much time with the baby.

Perhaps you were secretly hoping that your partner would choose to bottle-feed or would breastfeed for only a short time.

Perhaps you are very shy or easily embarrassed and feel uncomfortable when your partner breastfeeds in front of other people.

Perhaps you are concerned that breastfeeding is taking too much time.

The truth is that parenting takes time and energy no matter how you and your partner choose to feed your baby.

Managing negative feelings

So how do you manage negative feelings if they occur? You can begin by realizing that you play a greater role than anyone else in not just your partner's decision to breastfeed but also in her choice to continue breastfeeding. When a group of mothers was asked to name the one factor that most influenced their choice to breastfeed, 9 out of 10 mothers identified the feeding preference of their partner. That makes you a VIP (very important person) whether you realize it or not!

If you are comfortable talking with other new parents about your feelings, you may be surprised to learn that they have many of the same feelings. Some parents may even be willing to share tips on how to manage those feelings.

While breastfeeding may take more time during the early weeks than you had expected, it is still the best choice for your baby. If you are eager to feed your baby, just remember that the period of exclusive breastfeeding is only about 6 months (less than a football season!) and that when the time is right, you can be the first to offer solid foods. Even before 6 months, you can offer expressed (pumped) breast milk in a cup or bottle, depending on your baby's age and ability. If you offer a cup or bottle too soon, you can confuse your baby, so wait until your baby is breastfeeding well (at least 4–6 weeks after birth).

Parenting is never easy, so relax and enjoy this time together. Parenting a breastfed baby is a special joy, the benefits of which last a lifetime.

Remembering what you learned

The following list summarizes all the ways in which you can help to make breastfeeding the right choice for you and your partner.

- Learn as much as you can during pregnancy about the benefits of breastfeeding and the risks of not breastfeeding.

- Attend prenatal breastfeeding classes, childbirth classes, and parenting classes.

- Ask other parents about their breastfeeding experiences. Share your thoughts and feelings, and encourage them to do the same.

- Plan prenatal visits so that you can be present. Listen carefully to what the doctor says and ask questions. Get to know your baby before he is born.

- After your baby is born, watch others help with breastfeeding and ask them to show you how to help too.

- Learn how to diaper and bathe your baby.

- Limit visitors and the length of visits.

- Watch your baby closely for early signs of hunger such as sucking on fingers or fists, wiggling, and squirming. Bring your baby to your partner when it is time to breastfeed.

- Help your partner position your baby at the breast. Use extra pillows for support. Be sure that your partner is comfortable.

- Bring your partner water or juice and a healthy snack to eat while she breastfeeds.

- Stay close to your partner and keep her company while she breastfeeds. Let her know that you would like to burp and diaper your baby afterwards.

- Tell your partner what a wonderful mother she is and what a great job she is doing.

- Make a list of household chores that need to be done. Decide which chores you can do, and ask family and friends to help with others.

- Make dinner or dine in on takeout.

- Care for your baby for a period of time each day so that your partner can nap, bathe, read, or simply relax. Singing, dancing, or simply watching TV together gives you a chance to get to know your baby.

- Plan time alone with your partner. Ask someone you trust to care for your baby. Let your partner know that she is still an important part of your life.

- Keep your sense of humor—laughter is truly the best medicine!

- If your partner is returning to work outside the home, go shopping together to buy a breast pump and milk storage containers. Discuss various ways that you can make returning to work easier. See Chapter 11, "Breastfeeding and Working."

Babies change everything! They'll turn your life inside out and upside down. You will never be the person you were before. You will be a parent instead.

 Dads talk about what it's like to have a breastfed baby:

babygooroo.com/video/dads

Chapter 6

Especially for Teens

Are you going to breastfeed?

Chances are you have heard this question many times during your pregnancy. And you have probably discovered that some people have very strong feelings about breastfeeding, both good and bad, and are eager to share those feelings. Perhaps family and friends have already told you all the "facts" about breastfeeding?

   While it's true that family and friends can be a good source of information, if your family or friends did not breastfeed or found that breastfeeding was hard, they may not be the best source. Instead, you may want to ask your health care provider to introduce you to a mom who breastfed as a teen or, better yet, who is currently breastfeeding. An experienced mom knows firsthand the challenges that you will face as you try to balance school, work, friends, family, and motherhood!

Are my breasts too big or too small?

Will breastfeeding be painful?

How can I breastfeed after I go back to school?

Do I have to eat only healthy foods?

Can I smoke or drink alcohol if I breastfeed?

What if my boyfriend doesn't want me to breastfeed?

Can I use birth control?

The answers to these questions and more are found in this book and in the following stories from other teen moms. These are real stories from real moms.* And, just like you, they want to be the best mother that they can be.

Why should I breastfeed?

Breastfeeding is good for you and your baby! Babies who are breastfed are smarter and have better brain development. Children who were breastfed do better on IQ tests and often do better in school.

   Breastfed babies have fewer ear infections, less constipation and diarrhea, and less risk of childhood obesity. Breastfeeding, putting your baby on her back to sleep, and keeping your baby away from second-hand smoke all reduce your baby's risk of sudden infant death syndrome (SIDS). (See page 59 for suggestions on how to keep your baby safe from SIDS.)

   Breastfeeding protects you, too. Mothers who breastfeed have less bleeding after childbirth. They also have less risk of breast and ovarian cancer. This may not seem important now, but it can be important as you get older.

---

* I am most grateful to the people at Best Start Social Marketing for their kindness in allowing me to share these stories with you. The names of the mothers have been changed to protect their privacy.

What other teens say...

I believe, right now you are trying to decide if you should breastfeed or not. Just try it. If you find that you have problems, do not give up real quick. Call someone you know who has breastfed. Tell them you are having a problem. Talk it over with someone you trust. Clear your mind of all the advice, and all the wrong ideas you have been given about breastfeeding. Start fresh. Know that it is best for your baby to breastfeed and that you are going to do it.
—Kayla

Breastfed babies are less likely to get sick with stomach problems, ear infections, and colds. Breastfeeding keeps your baby healthy. Healthy babies are easier to take care of. It is easier for the mother and baby to breastfeed. —Latisha

It is easier to breastfeed. I don't have to make a bottle, and worry about boiling it or having the nipples ready. Breast milk is right there. It's always there. The milk doesn't spoil. It is so easy, simple, and fast and it is so good for the baby. It is the best thing for me and my baby. That's what I went with. —Hannah

Breastfeeding allows you to hold your baby in your arms and look into its eyes. This lets you feel all the love in the world. The way your baby looks at you will just melt your heart. —Jasmine

Is it hard to breastfeed?

Some people think that because breastfeeding is "natural" it must be easy. While making milk is natural, breastfeeding is a skill that you and your baby must learn.

Learning to breastfeed takes practice and patience. But once you learn, breastfeeding is easy.

What other teens say....

When I started breastfeeding I was real excited. But my baby did not want to take the breast at first. He rejected it a lot. The nurse said to be patient and he will do it. Then he breastfed fine.
—Tamika

How does breastfeeding make you feel?

Breastfeeding is the one thing that you can do for your baby that no one else can do. It is a good way to let family and friends know that you are this baby's mother and that the two of you have a special relationship.

Mothers who breastfeed have a special bond with their babies and are more confident in their ability to care for their babies.

What other teens say....

It gives me a proud feeling to breastfeed. An older woman walked up to me. She said, 'You know, I'm really proud of you because today you don't see young parents wanting to breastfeed their baby. They want to throw a bottle in their mouth and run out the door. But you are doing good.' She made me feel good. —Emma

It makes me feel proud to breastfeed. I am giving my daughter something no one else can give her. I help her survive. It makes me feel really good. —Shantell

I feel proud that I breastfeed. Many people said that I am too young to breastfeed. You are never too young. I mean, if you have a baby, you are not too young to breastfeed. —Lee

I like to breastfeed because I feel more mature. I feel like I am an adult because I have always been thought of as a child. Once I started breastfeeding, people stopped treating me like a child. It makes me feel more mature to breastfeed. —Niesha

I think it is just a general feeling that I get, because I know I'm giving something back to my baby. I watch her grow. It is really neat. I sit and think she is getting this from me. It is a great feeling. —Grace

Most people think that teens should not get pregnant. Well I did. It might have been a mistake. It might have been on purpose. But,

at least I am being careful to make sure my baby grows up healthy by breastfeeding. —Ava

How do I know if my baby is getting enough to eat?

Just remember, nothing comes out the bottom unless something goes in the top! As long as your baby has lots of poopy and wet diapers and is gaining the right amount of weight, you can be sure she is getting enough to eat.

If you are worried about your milk supply, talk with your baby's health care provider.

What other teens say....

That's why I like to breastfeed. I don't have to worry if my baby is getting enough to eat. I can breastfeed for as long as she wants to. As long as my baby has at least six wet diapers and four bowel movements a day, then I know she is getting enough breast milk. —Brianna

How will I survive with no sleep?

Breastfeeding saves time and energy, especially at night. There is no formula to mix, measure, and warm, so nighttime feedings are easier. Many mothers lie down to breastfeed at night so they can rest while their baby is feeding. Talk with your baby's health care provider about how to do this easily and safely.

What other teens say....

I decided to breastfeed so my baby would be healthy. Also, I don't have to carry bottles when I go places. I don't have to get up during the night to make bottles. —Jada

Doesn't breastfeeding tie you down?

Caring for a baby takes time, no matter how she is fed. Life is never simple, especially for busy teens, but breastfeeding can make life easier.

Breastfeeding mothers normally have one hand free to eat a meal, do homework, or talk on the telephone. Breasts and babies are portable, so mothers who breastfeed find it easier to come and go.

What other teens say....

It doesn't tie you down to breastfeed. It gives you more time with your baby. When you bottle-feed anyone can feed your baby. But when you breastfeed you have to spend time with your baby. So it gives you extra time to be with your baby and to bond with your baby. —Zoe

I think it makes the baby feel safe and secure to breastfeed and become more attached to me. My baby knows that I am his momma. It is not like my baby is going to be so hung up on me that I can't do anything. —Claire

Can I breastfeed if I have to go back to school?

Many teens (and even older mothers) continue to breastfeed after they go back to school. It just takes a little extra planning.

Be sure to read Chapter 11, "Breastfeeding and Working," since a lot of the information applies to mothers returning to school as well.

- Let your teachers know that you plan to continue breastfeeding. Because breastfed babies are healthier, mothers who breastfeed miss fewer days of school.

- Decide who will take care of your baby while you are away.

- If your child care provider is near the school, see if you can leave school to breastfeed during school hours.

- If you are unable to breastfeed during the day, your baby can be fed your expressed (pumped) milk or infant formula.

- If you plan to have expressed milk fed to your baby, you will need to learn how to express and store milk. See Chapter 9, "Expressing and Storing Your Milk."

- Ask your teachers or the school nurse to suggest a private place where you can express milk during school hours.

What other teens say....

Don't worry about having to go to school because you can still breastfeed in between. If you're just going to breastfeed at night, that's better than not breastfeeding at all. —Faith

What if my partner doesn't want me to breastfeed?

Talk with your partner about the benefits of breastfeeding for you and your baby. Encourage your partner to talk with other parents whose girlfriends or wives have breastfed. Help your partner separate breastfeeding facts from myths. Let your partner know how much you need their support as you learn to be a mother to your baby. Encourage your partner to spend time with your baby, too.

What other teens say....

After our baby was born, my boyfriend complained a lot when I breastfed our baby. It was like he had no part in it. He would go sit somewhere else, because I was not paying any attention to him. I told him to sit with me while I breastfed. This made him feel like he was more involved. Soon he got used to having me breastfeed. Now it's like a family thing. —Rebecca

You can pump your milk and have your boyfriend feed the baby, so he can also have that special bond with the baby. —Victoria

My husband wanted me to breastfeed, not just for the cost of it but for health, and he likes to watch me do it. —Madeline

When it is time to put the baby to sleep, the father can do that. Then he can have his own special time with the baby. —Sophia

Besides the bonding, it is much cheaper to breastfeed. It's just the natural thing to do. —Dwight

There is a real bond between the mother and child when they breastfeed. I see that bond between the two of them. Every mother should feel that bond. —Dylan

Can I use birth control?

If you are having sex but do not want to get pregnant, you will want to use some type of birth control. Talk with your partner and your health care provider about which type of birth control is best for you.

Nonhormonal methods include a diaphragm, sponge, intrauterine device (IUD), condom, and spermicidal cream, foam, or jelly. Hormonal methods include the pill, patch, shot, and ring. Hormonal methods that contain only progesterone are thought to be safe. Hormonal methods that contain estrogen can limit milk production.

If you decide to use a hormonal method, wait until your milk supply is well established (about 6 weeks after your baby's birth), and use a method that contains only progesterone. You may also want to stay away from the shot and use the pill, patch, or ring, which can be stopped easily if your milk supply goes down.

What other teens say....

If teens were taught ways to talk about sex with their partners before it happens, they'd make better decisions, either not having sex or having safer sex. —Acacia

Teens should also learn about contraception even if they don't plan on having sex. Be prepared, because you never know when something could change your mind … or your life. —Ashanti

Teens need to respect themselves and not be afraid to refuse sex without a condom or go to a clinic to get birth control. —Melissa

Since Laretha had the baby, we talk about birth control. I think the safest type of birth control for us at this time is to use the condom and the sponge. But whatever she chooses, I will support her. —Joseph

There are so many methods of birth control. It is always best to discuss the best type of birth control method with a doctor. —Anthony

Can I breastfeed in public?

You can breastfeed wherever you feel comfortable. Some mothers are shy at first about feeding in front of family or friends. But with a little practice, you can learn to breastfeed without your breasts showing.

Some new mothers like to practice in front of a mirror so they can see which clothing works best for breastfeeding in public.

If you are uncomfortable breastfeeding in public, you can always find a private place to breastfeed.

What other teens say....

There are no rules to breastfeeding. You can breastfeed wherever you feel comfortable. Don't worry about what other people think. Your baby needs to eat like everyone else. You should be able to feed your baby where you want to. —Maggie

For women who decide to breastfeed, do not let anyone tell you not to. —Deanna

Before I go into the store, I feed him in the car after we stop in the parking lot. Then he is real calm and quiet in the store. It's just better for me. But in a restaurant, I'll breastfeed him while our food is being prepared. By the time our food is ready, he is nice and quiet, so I can eat. —Kaitlyn

You can go anywhere, wherever you want you can go. I just put a blanket over me and my baby. Just cover up. I don't really care what people think. Breastfeeding is right for my baby and right for me. —Caroline

Can I breastfeed if I have small breasts?

Breasts come in all shapes and sizes. Breast size and shape do not affect your ability to make milk. But nipple size and shape can make breastfeeding easier or harder. Be patient. With a little practice, your baby will learn to breastfeed on your breasts.

With a little practice, you can learn to breastfeed without your breasts showing.

When you have a baby, the milk is there. If your breasts are small, you still have enough milk. It doesn't make any difference. Your chest could be the smallest in the world and your body will still make enough milk. —Geleen

Do I have to eat only healthy foods?

All mothers make healthy milk. While a healthy diet is best, mothers who eat "junk" food still produce enough milk to meet their baby's needs. Even if you prefer to eat "junk" food, try to also eat a variety of healthy foods each day, and drink enough so that you don't feel thirsty.

There are a few medicines you cannot take when you are breastfeeding. Before you take any medicine, even those sold over the counter (without a prescription), talk with your baby's health care provider to make sure that what you are taking is safe.

What other teens say....

I think it has been exaggerated that if you don't eat the right things you won't have enough milk. I try to eat good food, but there are times when I just can't fix a home-cooked meal. I have always had enough milk for my baby. Remember that what you eat and drink can be passed through your breast milk to your baby. Do not drink a lot of alcohol and do not take any medicines without talking to your doctor first. —Diedre

Your body will change naturally to make you hungrier and thirstier. This will help you eat enough to meet the extra needs required for milk production. Generally, if you're eating enough to feel full, your milk will have everything your baby needs for normal growth and development. —Yvonne

Very few people eat the right food all of the time. Eating junk foods and fast foods won't ruin your milk. Just remember that a variety of foods are needed for good health. Try to eat a balanced diet as often as possible. —Maria

What should I remember most?

Take one day at a time! Taking care of a new baby is hard work, so be proud of the job that you are doing. And remember that any amount of breastfeeding is good for you and your baby.

What other teens say....

That the breast is beautiful. It was placed on your body for a reason, not just for some man to hang on. Think about the way you feel. If it is right for you to breastfeed, then do it. And if it's not, there are other choices, but try to breastfeed first. —Isabella

Do not give up, if at first it doesn't seem to be going too well. It takes time to breastfeed. Even

if you only breastfeed for a few weeks, you will still have a beautiful experience to share with others. —Tara

Just like you, all of these young mothers and their partners are trying hard to give their babies the best start in life.

They hope that after hearing their stories, perhaps you will decide to breastfeed your baby, too!

HOW-TO'S

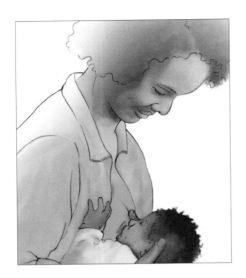

Chapter 7

Your First Breastfeeding

Ready or not, here he comes!

You know how the breast makes milk. Now you need to learn how to get the milk out of your breast and into your baby. With the excitement of your baby's birth, it is easy to forget what you have learned. So keep this book handy and take it with you to the hospital.

Your baby's first breastfeeding

Get to know your baby right away

If both you and your baby are healthy, hold your baby skin-to-skin between your breasts for at least the first hour after birth or ideally until your baby has breastfed for the first time. Babies are born with senses and reflexes that help them smell, crawl, lick, latch on, and breastfeed if given the chance—so lean back, relax, and let your baby take the lead. Expressing a few drops of colostrum may make it easier for your baby to find your breast. This first meeting is a learning experience for you and your baby, so relax and enjoy this time together.

Keep your baby with you day and night

Mothers and newborns should stay together (sharing a room 24 hours a day) whenever possible. When mothers and babies are together in the same room, learning to breastfeed is easier. Sharing a room also gives you and your baby a chance to get to know one another and allows you to practice your parenting skills while help is readily available. Mothers who share a room with their newborn actually get more rest than mothers who put their baby in a nursery at night.

Hold your baby skin-to-skin between your breasts
for at least the first hour after birth.

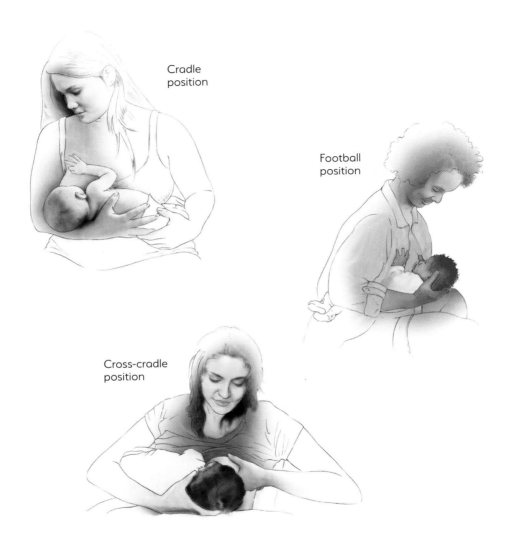

Cradle position

Football position

Cross-cradle position

Choose a breastfeeding position that is comfortable for you and your baby.
Use several different breastfeeding positions each day.

Side-lying
position

Reclining
position

Delay nonessential tasks

When your baby's first attempt at breastfeeding is delayed, learning to breastfeed can be more difficult. If possible, ask the hospital staff to wait at least 1 hour after your baby's birth, or until your baby breastfeeds for the first time, to do nonessential tasks such as diapering, bathing, and weighing.

Choose a comfortable position

The best breastfeeding positions are the ones that work for you and your baby. In the beginning, you may want to use the reclining (laid back) position, which allows your baby to locate your breast and latch on by himself (baby-led latch).

Once your baby is able to latch on and breastfeed well, you may prefer to sit up or lie on your side and bring your baby to your breast (mother-led latch). Regardless of which positions you choose, make sure your baby's chin, chest, and knees are facing your breast. Think about how you face the table to eat your meals, and position your baby the same way!

Moms share tips for positioning your baby:

babygooroo.com/video/positioning

Support and shape the breast

If you gently compress or shape your breast, it may be easier for your baby to latch on. Simply place your thumb and fingers opposite one another outside the areola and against your breast. Adjust the position of your thumb and fingers on your breast, so that the shaped breast lines up with the widest part of your baby's mouth in the same way that you would position a sandwich in front of your mouth. For example, a mother using the cradle position (baby lying on his side and facing the breast) would shape the breast using a U-hold (your hand is shaped like the letter U), while a mother using the football position (baby sitting up and facing the breast) would shape the breast using a C-hold (your hand is shaped like the letter C). If you prefer to use the V-hold, make sure your thumb and fingers are outside your areola.

Express (gently squeeze out) a few drops of colostrum

Express a few drops of colostrum before you offer your breast. If colostrum is readily available, your baby is more likely to latch on.

Tickle your baby's nose with your nipple

Babies are born with a "rooting reflex" that causes them to open their mouth and seek their mother's breast. You can trigger this reflex by gently rubbing your baby's cheek with your finger or your nipple. Choose the cheek closest to your breast. As your baby turns toward the breast, tickle his nose or his lips with your nipple until his mouth opens wide, as if he is yawning.

C-hold   U-hold   V-hold

Place your thumb and fingers outside the areola
to support and shape your breast.

Place your baby gently on your breast

Keeping your baby's head and shoulders in a straight line, position his lower lip and chin against your breast and gently bring him up and over your nipple and onto your breast. Again, think about how you position yourself for meals and position your baby the same way—facing the table. If your baby is positioned well, he is more likely to get a good, deep latch. Your nipple will point slightly toward the roof of your baby's mouth.

Do not lean forward. Bring your baby to you. When your baby is positioned correctly, his tongue should be over his lower gum, between his lower lip and the breast. His lips should curl out (not in) and lie flat against your breast. Hold your baby close, to prevent unnecessary pulling on your breast.

Check your areola (darker area around the nipple)

When your baby is positioned correctly, you may see little or none of the areola. How much you see will depend on the size of your areola and the size of your baby's mouth. You may notice that he is slightly off-center on the breast. As a result, you may see more areola on the top, above his lip, and less areola on the bottom.

Check your baby's nose, cheeks, and chin

Your baby's nose and cheeks may gently touch the breast. His chin should press firmly into the breast. Support his shoulders and back with your hand and arm. Place your

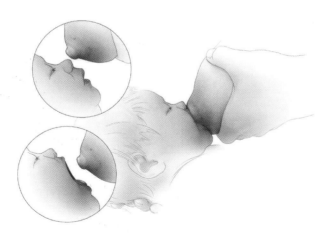

Wait for your baby to open his mouth wide,
then place him quickly but gently on the breast.

thumb and fingers below his ears and around the back of his neck. Babies breathe through their nose. If you place your hand on the back of your baby's head, you may press his nose into your breast and make breathing difficult.

If you have large breasts, you can gently lift the breast up from below with your fingers or place a rolled washcloth underneath your breast to let air enter your baby's nose. Do not press down on your breast with your thumb from above, or your nipple may slip out of your baby's mouth.

Break the suction

When your baby stops suckling and swallowing or falls asleep at the first breast, break the suction, burp him, wake him, and offer the second breast.

Break the suction before removing your baby from the breast.

You can break the suction by gently sliding your finger between your baby's gums and into his mouth. Protect your nipple with your finger as you take your baby off the breast.

Burp your baby

Breastfed babies usually take in less air than bottle-fed babies, so your baby may not burp after every feeding, but it is best to try. You may want to ask your partner to help.

Hold your baby upright in your lap or against your shoulder, or place him on his tummy across your lap. Be sure to have a clean cloth handy in case the burp is wet! Gently rub or pat his back. If he hasn't burped after a minute or two, you can offer the second breast.

Check your baby's position

You may feel a tugging sensation (some mothers describe it as a "painful" sensation) when your baby first latches on. However, the tugging sensation should stop once your baby draws your nipple and surrounding breast tissue into his mouth.

If the tugging sensation continues, remove your baby from the breast and try again.

Check your nipple

Your nipple will stretch out (lengthen) when your baby breastfeeds, but the shape of the nipple should look the same before and after he breastfeeds.

Some babies are unwilling to latch on well to the tissue around the nipple and latch on to the nipple instead. If your nipple is compressed between the roof of your baby's mouth above and his tongue below, your nipple will look flattened or creased and breastfeeding will be painful! If the pain lasts more than a few seconds, break the suction, remove your baby from your breast, and try again.

Use a breast pump if needed

If your nipples are flat or inverted and your baby is unable to maintain a good, deep latch, you may want to use a breast pump before each breastfeeding to gently pull your nipple out.

Choose a hand pump, battery-operated pump, or electric pump, whichever is readily available. Adjust the suction control to the lowest setting, center your nipple in the opening (flange), and apply gentle suction for 5–10 seconds.

If necessary, release the suction and repeat the action. As soon as your nipple moves out, remove the pump and quickly put your baby on your breast.

Try different positions for burping to see which ones work best.

Your baby's next breastfeedings

Keep your baby with you day and night

It may be several hours before your baby wakes to breastfeed again. Many babies breastfeed early and often, but others may show little interest in breastfeeding at first. Keep your baby with you day and night while you are in the hospital and also during the first few weeks at home.

Look and listen for early signs of hunger or light sleep such as squirming, lip-smacking, or finger-sucking, and offer your breast at those times.

Breastfeed at least eight times in each 24-hour period

Breastfed babies need only small amounts of breast milk at first. Small, frequent feedings give you and your baby a chance to practice breastfeeding while help is available. They also make it easier for your baby to adjust to life outside your body. Last but not least, frequent feedings lead to frequent bowel movements, resulting in lower levels of bilirubin and less risk for jaundice.

During the first day or two, a breastfed baby eats about 1–1½ teaspoons (5–7 ml) of breast milk at each feeding. As your baby grows, so does your milk supply. By the end of

Day 1
1–1½ teaspoons
(5–7 ml)
at each feeding

Day 3
¾–1¼ ounces
(23–38 ml)
at each feeding

Day 7
2–2½ ounces
(60–75 ml)
at each feeding

Moms share tips on how to know your baby is hungry:

babygooroo.com/video/hungry

the first week, your baby will be eating about 2–2½ ounces (60–75 ml) at a feeding.

Some babies breastfeed regularly day and night. Others cluster-feed, breastfeeding every hour for three to five feedings, then sleeping for several hours in between clusters. Every baby is different! Your baby will let you know when she is hungry. If you keep your baby nearby, you won't miss those early feeding cues. Supplements are seldom necessary unless your baby continues to lose weight.

Wake a sleepy baby

Sometimes a sleepy baby will not ask to eat often enough. During the first few weeks, if your baby does not wake to breastfeed at least eight times in each 24 hours, place her skin-to-skin between your breasts. Watch for early signs of hunger or light sleep and offer your breast at those times. Other tips for waking a sleepy baby include:

- dimming the lights

- unwrapping her

- changing her diaper

- washing her bottom with a warm washcloth

- massaging her feet (my favorite!)

- placing her in your lap in a sitting position, supporting her chin in one hand and massaging her back with the other hand

Relieve fullness and prevent engorgement

Your milk supply will increase greatly about 3–5 days after birth. Your breasts may feel firm and full. Frequent feedings will relieve fullness and prevent engorgement.

Breastfeed at least eight times in each 24-hour period.

If necessary, hand express or pump to soften your breasts and relieve the fullness.

Continue to position your baby correctly on your breast

You might feel soreness (pain) when your baby first latches on. However, the soreness should stop as she draws your nipple and the surrounding breast tissue into her mouth. If the soreness continues, remove your baby from the breast and try again.

Remember that when your baby is positioned correctly, her head and chest should be facing your breast. Her mouth should be opened wide. Her tongue should be over her lower gum, between her lower lip and the breast. Her lips should curl out (not in), and lie flat against your breast. Her nose and cheeks may gently touch your breast. Her chin should press firmly into your breast.

Moms share tips on how to know your baby has a good latch:

babygooroo.com/video/latch

You may see little or none of your areola. The amount you see will depend on the size of your areola and the size of your baby's mouth.

Know the signs of poor latch

To transfer milk, your baby must latch on to your breast correctly. When your baby is positioned correctly, your nipple and the surrounding breast tissue will fill your baby's mouth. Your nipple should be at the back of her mouth, with little or no pressure on the nipple itself. Your nipple should look the same before and after you breastfeed. When your baby is positioned incorrectly, nipple pain and damage can occur. Signs of a poor latch include:

- nipples that are flattened or creased after breastfeeding

- clicking sounds by your baby while breastfeeding

- dimpling of your baby's cheeks while breastfeeding

- pain while breastfeeding or between feedings

Know the signs of milk transfer

When your baby is positioned correctly, the milk ducts (located beneath the areola) are drawn into your baby's mouth and compressed between the roof of her mouth above and her tongue below, forming a sandwich.

The sudden release of milk from the breasts is called the let-down reflex or milk-ejection reflex. Most mothers have more than one let-down per feeding. You may feel a tingling or fullness in your breasts when your milk lets down, or you may notice milk leaking from one breast while your baby breastfeeds from the opposite breast. Don't be concerned if you see or feel nothing; every mother is different. Simply watch your baby. Look and listen for signs of swallowing. When your milk lets down, your baby's sucking pattern will change from short, rapid sucks to a slower, rhythmic, suckle-swallow pattern.

Watch your baby, not the clock

Breastfeed as long as your baby wishes on the first breast before you offer the second breast. This is called *baby-led feeding*.

When your baby stops suckling and swallowing or falls asleep at the first breast, break the suction, burp her, wake her, and offer the second breast.

If you limit the frequency or the length of feedings, your baby may not get the calories and nutrients she needs to grow. So follow your baby's lead and breastfeed at the first sign of hunger and continue to breastfeed until your baby is satisfied.

Offer both breasts at each feeding

Offer both breasts at each feeding, but do not be concerned if your baby seems satisfied with one breast. Each breast can provide a full meal.

If your baby breastfeeds poorly on the first breast and shows no sign of suckling and swallowing, offer the first breast again.

If necessary, hand express or pump to relieve fullness in the second breast.

Begin each feeding on the breast offered last

For the next feeding, begin on the breast offered last and alternate the beginning breast with each new feeding. This will ensure that both breasts get equal stimulation.

Watch your baby, not the clock.

Support your baby well

Support your baby well in whatever positions you choose. This will prevent unnecessary pulling on your breast, keep your baby positioned correctly, and prevent nipple soreness.

Avoid pacifiers and artificial nipples

Bottle nipples and pacifiers, if used too soon, can confuse your baby. Once you and your baby have learned to breastfeed well (about 3–4 weeks after birth), you can begin to offer a pacifier at naptime and bedtime in order to reduce your baby's risk of sudden infant death syndrome (SIDS). A pacifier coated with sugar water can also be used for pain relief during painful procedures such as heel sticks or injections (shots).

Avoid water or formula supplements

Your milk provides all the nutrients your baby needs for about the first 6 months. Frequent use of water or formula supplements can decrease your milk supply and lead to early weaning (stopping breastfeeding).

If giving a supplement is necessary for medical reasons, choose a method of supplementation that is least likely to interfere with your baby's ability to breastfeed later. For example, you can supplement at the breast with a supplemental feeding device or with a feeding tube and syringe, or you can supplement away from the breast using a spoon, eye dropper, or cup. If you decide to use a bottle with an artificial nipple, choose a soft, supple nipple with a wide base and a slow flow.

Keep a daily log

During the first 2–4 weeks, while you and your baby are learning to breastfeed, you may want to keep a daily log of your baby's breastfeedings, wet diapers, and bowel movements (poops).

Knowing what to expect during the early weeks will give you confidence in your ability to breastfeed and let you know when to seek help.

- Expect at least eight breastfeedings in each 24 hours.

- Expect clear or pale yellow urine and six or more wet diapers a day by day 5.

- After day 1, expect at least three stools a day for the next 4 weeks.

- Your baby's stools will be black and sticky (meconium) on days 1 and 2, green and pasty on days 3 and 4, and yellow, seedy, and runny by day 5.

- If your baby has black stools on day 3, green stools on day 5, or fewer stools than expected, call your baby's health care provider right away.

Daily log of your baby's breastfeedings, wet diapers, and bowel movements (poops).

DAY	BREASTFEEDINGS (8 OR MORE)	WET DIAPERS (6 OR MORE)	POOPS (3 OR MORE)
EXAMPLE	̶H̶t̶ ̶H̶t̶ I	̶H̶t̶ I	IIII
MONDAY			
TUESDAY			
WEDNESDAY			
THURSDAY			
FRIDAY			
SATURDAY			
SUNDAY			

- Expect small, frequent, runny stools with very little solid material. Sometimes, all you see in the diaper is a yellow stain the size of your baby's fist.

- Breastfed babies' stools look like a mixture of water, yellow mustard, cottage cheese, and sesame seeds!

- After the first 4–6 weeks, expect larger and fewer stools. Many babies have one large stool every 1–5 days, though others continue to have small, frequent stools each day for many months.

Keep track of your baby's weight

Your baby's health care provider will weigh your baby during each health check.

- Expect your baby to lose no more than 7 percent of her birth weight.

- After the first week, expect your baby to gain at least 5 ounces each week during the first 3 months.

Number and color of stools during the first month.

DAY	NUMBER	COLOR
1	1+	Black
2	3+	Black
3	3+	Green
4	3+	Green
5–28	3+	Yellow

Moms share tips on how to tell your baby is getting enough to eat:

babygooroo.com/video/enough

Chapter 8

Continuing to Breastfeed

Congratulations! You made it!

During the first weeks after birth your focus should be on taking care of yourself and your baby. Which means leaving household chores to others—cooking and cobwebs can wait! Nap at least once a day when your baby naps, and wear your pajamas or nightgown during the first week as a reminder to family and friends that you are still recovering from pregnancy, labor, and birth. Accept all offers of help, and don't hesitate to ask for help. The frustrations of parenting seem greater when parents are worn out from too little sleep.

If necessary, limit visitors and the length of visits. Place a small "Do Not Disturb" sign on the front door to discourage unwanted guests.

Though some mothers are comfortable breastfeeding in front of family and friends (both male and female), many are not. It is important that you be relaxed. So don't hesitate to speak up if you need more privacy.

Though it is nice to have help at home, family and friends can be a source of stress if their knowledge of breastfeeding is limited. You may need to explain politely the benefits of breastfeeding and the importance of frequent feedings, feeding on request, and nighttime feedings. Explain that it is better for you and your baby to nap during the day and breastfeed at night than for Grandma to bottle-feed your baby so that you can sleep through the night.

Eat a variety of healthy foods, and drink to satisfy your thirst. If your urine is clear or pale yellow in color, you will know that you are drinking enough fluid. Use each breastfeeding as a reminder to eat a light snack or drink a beverage. You can begin light exercise 2–4 weeks after birth. However, listen to what your body tells you. Many mothers, eager to resume their active lifestyles, do too much too soon and quickly regret it. Remember, these early weeks are a learning experience for the whole family, so relax and enjoy this time together.

The "baby blues" and postpartum depression

After your baby is born, you may find that you feel happy one minute and sad the next. You may even cry for no clear reason. These are signs of the "baby blues." The baby blues are common and usually occur 3 to 4 days after birth and last several days.

If your symptoms last longer or grow worse, you may have a more serious illness called *postpartum depression*. Postpartum depression can occur right after birth, or weeks or months later. Signs of postpartum depression include:

- not wanting to care for yourself or for your baby

- loss of appetite

- no energy

- trouble sleeping

- feeling sad or guilty

- feeling anxious or scared

- feeling angry

- thinking of hurting yourself or your baby

No one knows what causes postpartum depression. Hormone changes that occur during pregnancy and after birth were thought to play a role, but there is little evidence to support that theory.

Postpartum depression can last for several weeks or many months. It's important to know that postpartum depression doesn't last forever. If you are feeling overwhelmed, that's okay. Birth brings many changes, and parenting isn't easy. The sooner you get help, the sooner you will feel better.

The following is a list of things you can do that other mothers with postpartum depression have found helpful.

- Find someone to talk to, and tell that person how you feel.

- Be honest about what you can and cannot do, and ask others for help. Do not try to be *supermom*.

- Get help with child care and household chores.

- Do something for yourself each day, even if it's for only 10 or 15 minutes. Reading, exercising (walking is good for you and easy to do), taking a bath, or listening to music are good choices.

- Accept that you may get only one thing done each day. There may be days when you can't get anything done. Try not to get angry with yourself when this happens.

- Write down your thoughts and feelings each day. Once you begin to feel better, reread what you wrote. It will help you see that you are getting better.

- Find a support group in your area. Accept all offers of help!

- Talk with your health care provider about your feelings. She can offer counseling and/or medicine. If you are concerned about taking an antidepressant, it may help to know that the benefits of breastfeeding often outweigh the possible risks of antidepressants. Some antidepressants, however, are safer than others, so be sure to talk with your doctor about which medicine is best for you and your baby.

It's important to remember that postpartum depression is an illness, not a weakness, and like other illnesses, it needs to be treated. Most treatments, including the use of antidepressants, are safe for breastfeeding mothers and babies. Talk with your health care provider about the treatment that is best for you. Some studies show that breastfeeding may actually lessen the symptoms of postpartum depression. So every effort should be made to preserve this special relationship between you and your baby.

Getting to know your breastfed baby

Every baby has basic needs—food, oxygen, warmth, safety, and love. You will know your baby's needs are met if you understand how normal breastfed babies behave. If you have family members or friends who have breastfed, watching them with their babies may have taught you a lot about newborn behavior. But if the mothers you know have not breastfed, or have breastfed for only a short time, you may have much to learn.

During the first 3 months, babies grow fast, which explains why they need lots of calories. Since your baby's stomach is about the size of his fist, it is easy to understand why he needs to eat often (at least eight times in each 24 hours). Watch your baby for early signs of hunger and offer the breast at those times. If you offer your breast while your baby is quiet but alert, he is more likely to latch on and breastfeed well. Crying is the last sign of hunger and should be avoided. If your baby has to cry to be fed, he is more likely to breastfeed poorly or fall asleep at the breast after only a minute or two.

You can be sure that your baby is getting enough to eat if he has small, frequent poops (three or more each day), heavy, wet diapers (six or more each day), and steady weight gain (at least 5 ounces each week).

Once your baby is breastfeeding well and gaining weight, you can begin to let him set his own feeding schedule. This may happen about 4–6 weeks after birth. But remember that every baby is different. Some babies will continue to breastfeed day and night for many weeks. Other babies will breastfeed every 1–2 hours when awake and sleep for longer periods of time in between.

If your baby sleeps for 3 hours or more at a time during the early weeks, you may need to express enough milk to relieve fullness, prevent engorgement, and maintain your milk supply. Expressed breast milk can be stored in the refrigerator or freezer for later use. As your baby's feeding pattern changes, your breasts will respond to your baby's changing needs and will make just the right amount of milk. Breasts truly are amazing!

If my baby has colic, can I still breastfeed?

Colic—long periods of fussing and crying each day for no clear reason—occurs in 10–20 percent of newborns. Colic occurs in formula-fed babies as well as in breastfed babies. The symptoms usually appear 2–6 weeks after birth and disappear by 12–16 weeks of age. The cause of colic is unclear. Occasionally, overfeeding or something in the infant's or the mother's diet can cause fussiness. More often no cause is found.

If your baby cries nonstop for hours, try offering one breast at each feeding. The result will be a low-volume, low-sugar, high-fat meal. In addition, avoid giving your baby formula containing cow's milk, and avoid consuming milk products, eggs, nuts, and wheat yourself. See Chapter 17, "Breastfeeding and Allergies."

Constant sounds or vibrations from a vacuum cleaner, clothes dryer, car engine, untuned television, or white noise machine may soothe a fussy baby. A warm compress on your baby's abdomen can also be helpful. A warm tub bath, a warm washcloth, or a warm water bottle works well. While colic seldom lasts more than 16 weeks, it can seem like 16 years! A mother unable to calm her baby feels guilty. A partner unable to calm a mother feels helpless. If the fussiness continues, your baby's doctor can prescribe medicine.

Weaning is seldom necessary. Frequently, the use of infant formula makes the symptoms worse. As your infant's intestinal tract matures, the symptoms will improve. While infants in some cultures cry off and on for 2–3 hours a day, in cultures where babies are carried in slings throughout the day, colic is rarely seen.

The American Academy of Pediatrics recommends that mothers and babies sleep near one another but on separate sleep surfaces.

When will my baby sleep through the night?

It's important to remember that every baby is different. Between 6 and 12 weeks of age, many babies will begin to sleep for 4–5 hours at night, while others will continue to breast-feed regularly throughout the night. As long as your baby is growing well, you can try to lengthen the amount of time between feedings at night by diapering, walking, and rocking. Many babies sleep for 6 hours at night starting around 6 months of age. As your baby gets older, he will sleep for a longer period of time at night. However, your definition of "night" will need to change!

Where your baby sleeps is also important. Babies often sleep in more than one place, including car seats, cribs, cots, bassinets, co-sleepers (baby beds that attach to the side of adult beds), and adult beds. While some sleep areas are safe, others are not.

The American Academy of Pediatrics (AAP) recommends that mothers and babies sleep near one another but on separate sleep surfaces. When mothers and babies sleep near one another, nighttime feedings are easier, babies breastfeed more often, and mothers get more sleep. Babies who breastfeed more often have fewer periods of deep sleep. Less time spent in deep sleep may lower your baby's risk of sudden infant death syndrome (SIDS), the leading cause of death in children between 1 month and 1 year of age.

The following suggestions will help you and your baby sleep safely.

- Place your baby on his back to sleep. Do not place your baby on his tummy or on his side. If your baby has a medical condition that prevents him from sleeping on his back, talk with your baby's doctor about a safe sleeping position.

- Place your baby on a firm mattress or other firm surface to sleep.

- Do not place your baby on sofas or overstuffed chairs to sleep.

- Do not place your baby in an adult bed to sleep.

- Do not place your baby in an adult bed with older siblings to sleep.

- Use only a lightweight cover or blanket in your baby's bed, or place your baby in a sleep sack. Do not use a comforter, duvet, quilt, or pillow.

- Keep your baby comfortable. Do not let your baby get too hot. Use a single layer of clothing in addition to his diaper.

- Keep your baby in a smoke-free place for at least the first year of his life.

- Take your baby for regular health checks and immunizations.

- Call your baby's doctor right away if your baby seems sick.

What are growth spurts?

Growth spurts usually occur around 1, 3, and 6 weeks of age, but can happen at any time. Your baby may be fussy and restless and want to breastfeed all the time. Well-meaning but inexperienced friends and relatives may suggest that "your milk isn't rich enough," that "you're not making enough milk," that "your baby needs infant formula or solid foods," or that "it is time to stop breastfeeding."

Take a deep breath and relax. After 2–3 days of more frequent breastfeedings, your milk supply will catch up with the increased demand, and the length and frequency of breastfeedings will decrease.

What are nursing strikes?

A nursing strike is a sudden refusal by your baby to breastfeed. It can last for several hours or for several days. Sometimes there is a clear cause such as teething, fever, ear infection, stuffy nose, or constipation. Occasionally, menstruation (monthly bleeding) or something in your diet will change the taste of your milk. Deodorant, perfume, or lotion placed on your skin may cause a strike, but frequently no cause is found.

If you experience a nursing strike, simply hand express or pump your breasts until the strike ends. In the meantime, feed your baby your expressed milk using a teaspoon, eye dropper, medicine spoon, or cup. Continue to offer your breast, but don't insist. Choose a quiet place where you can give your baby your undivided attention. Last but not least, don't panic! Nursing strikes seldom lead to weaning.

How can I keep my baby from getting a flat head?

- Your baby's brain needs room to grow, so her head is made up of soft bones that grow together over time. When babies spend a lot of time on their backs, a flat spot can form on their heads, and little or no hair may grow on that spot. This condition is called plagiocephaly, a fancy word that means flat head.

- Premature babies are more likely to get a flat spot on their heads because their heads are even softer than those of full-term babies. You can prevent flat spots on your baby's head by holding your baby skin-to-skin against your chest, a technique known as kangaroo care. While it's important to put your baby on her back to sleep in order

Place your baby on her tummy while she is awake to help prevent a flat head.

to reduce the risk of sudden infant death syndrome (SIDS), you can protect your baby's head by placing her on her stomach when she is awake (tummy time) or carrying her upright in a sling. Tummy time will also strengthen the muscles needed for crawling and sitting. Because the risk of SIDS is greater when babies are on their tummies, never leave your baby alone during tummy time.

Can I breastfeed in public?

In the United States, women who breastfeed in public sometimes get dirty looks or hear nasty comments. As a result, in many states there are laws protecting a woman's right to breastfeed wherever she has the right to be.

If you are shy or easily embarrassed, you may want to choose a private place where you will not be disturbed and wear clothing that makes it easier to breastfeed without being noticed. If you choose to breastfeed in public, know that in doing so, you will encourage other mothers to do the same.

Do I need to give my baby vitamins?

The American Academy of Pediatrics (AAP) recommends that all newborns be given a single injection (shot) of vitamin K soon after birth. Vitamin K reduces your baby's risk of bleeding by helping his blood to clot. A shot of vitamin K protects your baby until the bacteria in her bowel (gut) start to make vitamin K.

The AAP also recommends that all breastfed babies be given a daily dose of vitamin D. Vitamin D builds healthy bones and reduces your baby's risk of rickets. The main source of vitamin D is the sun. However, too much sun exposure can be harmful, so the AAP recommends that breastfed babies be given 400 IU of vitamin D each day beginning soon after birth. Liquid vitamins are available at most grocery stores and drugstores. Follow the package directions to make sure your baby gets the right amount of vitamin D each day.

Iron is a mineral that carries oxygen in the blood. During the last weeks of pregnancy, babies store enough iron in their livers to meet their iron needs for about 6 months. After 6 months, babies rely on iron-rich foods such as red meat, dark poultry, egg yolks, beans, and iron-fortified cereal and pasta. If your baby's iron level is low, her health care provider may recommend an iron supplement.

Moms share tips on breastfeeding away from home:

babygooroo.com/video/public

Chapter 9

Expressing and Storing Your Milk

Milk expression, like breastfeeding, is a learned skill. And like any new skill, it takes patience and practice. If you are uncertain about when to express, simply watch your breasts, not the clock! Express whenever your breasts feel full or whenever it is convenient.

How often you express milk will depend upon your needs and the needs of your baby. For example, if you or your baby is unable to breastfeed for health reasons, you may need to express throughout the day and at night. If you need to be away from your baby for a period of time each day, you may need to express one or more times a day. But if you and your baby are seldom apart, you may need to express only once or twice a week.

As long as you have a good supply of milk, your breasts will tell you when you need to express. But if your milk supply is low, you may need to express more often to increase your supply. Breast milk can be collected by hand expression, hand pump, battery-operated pump, or electric pump. Mothers who plan to pump now and then will find that hand expression, a hand pump, a battery-operated pump, or a semi-automatic electric pump works well. Mothers who need to pump daily or for many weeks or months may want to rent or purchase a fully automatic electric pump.

Even if you choose to use a breast pump, you should still learn to hand express. Hand expression combined with pumping removes more of the available milk, and mothers who combine the two often produce more milk.

Your first tries at expressing your milk may produce only enough milk to cover the bottom of the collection container. Don't get discouraged. It may take several days or weeks before you see an increase in the amount of milk obtained.

In the beginning you may want to express and collect from one breast while your baby breastfeeds from the opposite breast. Infant suckling will stimulate a let-down reflex and increase the flow of milk. As your confidence grows, you may want to express milk early in the morning or between feedings when your breasts seem full. It is important that you relax and think about your baby. This will encourage milk release and increase the amount of milk obtained.

Pumping one breast while your baby breastfeeds on the opposite breast can increase the amount of milk expressed.

Hand expressing

- Choose a quiet, comfortable place where you will not be disturbed. If necessary, silence your phone and lock the door. Gather all of your supplies together, including a healthy snack and drink for yourself.

- Use a container with a wide opening. A mayonnaise or peanut butter jar works best. Choose a container that has been washed in hot, soapy water and rinsed well, or cleaned in a dishwasher.

- Wash your hands with soap and water and rinse well. Putting warm water on your breasts can make expression easier. Warm washcloths or a shower or bath works well.

- Gently massage the breasts in a circular pattern using the flat part of your fingers. Roll your nipple between your thumb and finger. This can cause a let-down reflex and make milk expression easier.

- Relax and think about your baby. This can help milk release and increase the amount of milk obtained. Looking at a picture of your baby, holding something he has worn, or listening to music or relaxing sounds can also be helpful.

- Gently support your breast with one or both hands. Place your thumb and first two fingers opposite each other on your breast, about 1–2 inches from the base of the nipple.

- Press in toward your chest, then slowly bring your thumb and fingers together, compressing your breast between your thumb and fingers. Do not squeeze hard or pinch. Do not compress the nipple itself.

- Change the position of your thumb and fingers on your breast and repeat the press and compress motion until all parts of your breast have been expressed and the flow of milk slows down. Think of your breast as the face of a clock. Place your thumb and fingers at the 6 o'clock and 12 o'clock positions, then at 1 and 7, 2 and 8, and 3 and 9.

- Repeat the procedure on the opposite breast. Express each breast several times until the desired amount of milk has been collected,

Rotate the placement of your thumb and fingers on the breast until all parts of the breast are soft and the flow of milk slows down.

the flow of milk slows down, or your breasts feel soft. Refrigerate or freeze your milk for later use. See pages 68–72 for storage guidelines.

- As with breastfeeding, patience and practice are the keys to success.

Expressing with a breast pump

- Choose a quiet, comfortable place where you will not be disturbed. If necessary, silence your phone and lock the door. Gather all of your supplies together, including a healthy snack and drink for yourself.

- Wash your hands with soap and water and rinse well.

- Gently massage your breasts in a circular pattern using the flat part of your fingers. Roll your nipple between your thumb and fingers. This can cause a let-down reflex and make milk expression easier.

- Relax and think about your baby. This can help milk release and increase the amount of milk obtained. Looking at a picture of your baby, holding something he has worn, or listening to music or relaxing sounds can also be helpful.

- Adjust the suction control of the breast pump to the lowest setting. Center your

nipple in the opening. Follow the directions that come with the pump.

- It may take several minutes for milk to flow. Pump until the flow of milk slows to a drip. If you are pumping both breasts at the same time, rest for several minutes, then repeat once or twice. If you are pumping one breast at a time, you can switch back and forth from breast to breast and do not need to wait. You can slowly increase the suction as long as you are comfortable. With double-pumping you may find that one breast softens before the other, and you may still need to massage and single-pump the other breast or hand express in order to relieve the fullness.

- Express each breast several times until the desired amount of milk has been collected or your breasts feel soft. Watch your breasts and the flow of milk rather than the clock. Refrigerate or freeze your milk for later use. The collection container that comes with a pump can often be used for storage.

- Wash the collection kit after each use in hot, soapy water and rinse well. During work hours, rinse the collection kit in hot water and wash in hot, soapy water when you get home.

- As with breastfeeding, patience and practice are the keys to success.

Choosing a breast pump

The best pump is the one that works for you!

Some mothers rent or purchase a breast pump during their last weeks of pregnancy so that they will be ready for their return to work. But once you hold your baby in your arms, you may find that plans made during pregnancy change. For example, you may end up working fewer hours and pumping less than you had planned. So consider waiting until after your baby is born to choose a breast pump.

Pumps can be rented or purchased from hospitals, pump rental stations, and medical supply companies. Check with your baby's doctor, your lactation consultant, or your nurse for the location nearest your home. The following information will help you choose a pump that is right for you.

Types of pumps

Different types of breast pumps are available to satisfy every need.

Hand pump

There are many types of hand pumps. It's important to choose one that you find easy to use.

You need two hands to use some hand pumps and only one hand to use others. Many mothers choose hand pumps because they are inexpensive and readily available. While some hand pumps work quite well, others offer poor suction and poor milk removal.

Battery-operated pump

Battery-operated pumps are powered by one or more batteries. The type of battery varies from pump to pump. As the battery power decreases, the strength of the suction decreases as well. Some battery-operated pumps have AC adapters that limit the need for batteries.

Some mothers like battery-operated pumps because only one hand is needed to operate the pump. But battery replacement can be very costly if the pump is used often. You can use rechargeable batteries, but they often produce less suction than alkaline batteries.

Semi-automatic electric pump

Semi-automatic electric pumps create constant suction. To release the suction, you must cover and uncover a small hole in the base of the flange. Too much suction can damage nipples, so care must be taken to release the suction regularly.

Fully automatic electric pump

Fully automatic electric pumps routinely cycle the amount of suction produced. This limits the risk of nipple damage and increases the amount of milk expressed. In addition, fully automatic electric pumps have both single and double collection kits so that you can pump one or both breasts at a time.

Factors to consider

Factors to consider in choosing a breast pump include:

- reason for use (to increase milk supply, establish a milk supply, provide an occasional supplement, or feed a preterm infant)

- frequency of use

- effectiveness

- comfort

- ease of operation and cleaning

- availability

- durability

- cost

Features to look for include:

- pressure range and suction control

- flange size and shape

- storage capacity

- backflow protection

Flanges are made out of silicone, soft or hard plastic, or glass. They come in different sizes to fit a variety of nipples and breasts. If necessary an insert can be placed inside the flange to improve the fit.

Many pumps have special parts that fit inside the pump and prevent the flow of expressed milk into the motor or battery case (backflow).

If you plan to pump now and then (once or twice a week), you should consider hand expression, a hand pump, a battery-operated pump, or a semi-automatic electric pump. Hand pumps and battery-operated pumps need to be purchased rather than rented.

A fully automatic electric pump comes with a double collection kit that lets you pump both breasts at once, saving time and energy.

If you would like to be able to pump one breast while your baby breastfeeds from the opposite breast, you should consider a squeeze-handle hand pump, a battery-operated pump, or a semi-automatic electric pump. All of these pumps can be operated easily with one hand.

If you plan to pump frequently (one or more times a day) or for many weeks or months, you may want to rent or purchase a fully automatic electric pump.

A fully automatic electric pump comes with a double collection kit that lets you pump both breasts at once, saving time and energy. In addition, double-pumping increases prolactin levels, which increases milk production.

Store your milk in any container made for food.

Most breast pumps are designed to be used by only one person (single-user pumps), but some fully automatic electric pumps can be used by more than one person (multiple-user pumps). Pumps that are used in the hospital (hospital-grade pumps) or are available for rent must be able to be used safely by more than one person. Multiple-user pumps can be cleaned completely to ensure that the breast milk of one mother does not come into contact with the breast milk of another mother.

The table on the following page will help you identify a method of milk expression that will help you achieve your specific breastfeeding goal.

Storing your milk

Confused about how long to store your expressed milk? You're not alone. Even well-respected health care organizations don't always agree on how long breast milk can be safely stored.

So what's a mother to do? Keep it simple. Handle your milk the same way you care for other foods. Store your milk in a cool place, refrigerate it as soon as possible, and freeze it for later use. Because storage time and temperature can affect the nutrients in breast milk, follow these simple guidelines:

• Store your milk in any glass or BPA-free container made for food.

• Place a single serving in each container.

Methods of milk expression that meet specific breastfeeding goals.

GOAL	HAND EXPRESSION	HAND PUMP	BATTERY-OPERATED PUMP	SEMI-AUTOMATIC ELECTRIC PUMP	FULLY AUTOMATIC ELECTRIC PUMP
To begin a milk supply					x
To increase a milk supply	x	x	x	x	x
To provide an occasional supplement	x	x	x		
To provide human milk for a hospitalized preterm infant					x
To pump one or two times a week	x	x	x	x	
To pump one or more times a day or for many weeks or months					x
To pump while your baby breastfeeds from the opposite breast		x (squeeze-handle models)	x	x	
To double-pump				x	x

- Label the container with your baby's name, the date, and the time.

- If you plan to freeze your milk, don't forget to allow room for expansion.

During the first 1–6 months, healthy, full-term babies eat about 25 ounces each day. You can estimate the size of a single serving by dividing your baby's total daily intake (25 ounces) by the number of feedings. For example 25 ounces divided by 8 feedings equals approximately 3 ounces per serving.

You can combine small amounts of expressed breast milk collected throughout the day to make a single serving.

Storage recommendations vary and are often based on studies done under ideal conditions in which mothers have access to clean equipment and a cool room. Real-life conditions, however, are often less than ideal. The Special Supplemental Nutrition Program for Women, Infants and Children (WIC) recommends that freshly expressed breast milk be stored at room temperature for up to 4 hours, in the refrigerator for up to 4 days, and in the freezer section of a refrigerator for up to 6 months.

Store breast milk in the back of the refrigerator or freezer, away from the door.

To thaw, place the unopened container in the refrigerator or in a pan of warm water. Do not thaw or warm breast milk in a microwave oven. A microwave destroys live cells and heats the milk unevenly, which increases the risk of burning your baby.

Breast milk can be served chilled from the refrigerator or at room temperature. No heating is necessary. If your baby prefers milk at room temperature, simply place the unopened container in a pan of warm water for several minutes.

Milk that has been thawed in the refrigerator should be used within 4 hours after it is removed from the refrigerator or within 24 hours if it is kept in the refrigerator. Milk that has been thawed in a pan of warm water should be used right away or stored in the refrigerator for up to 2 hours.

Milk left in the feeding container (e.g., bottle or cup) can be stored in the refrigerator and used within 2 hours to complete the feeding.

Label each bottle of breast milk with your baby's name, the date, and the time.

Learn more about how to store your milk:

babygooroo.com/handouts

Room (refrigerate as soon as possible)
Up to 4 hours at 77°F (25°C) or colder

Refrigerator
Up to 4 days at 40°F (4°C) or colder

Freezer section
Up to 6 months at 0°F (-18°C) or colder

Breast milk storage guidelines for healthy, full-term babies.

Source: U.S. Department of Agriculture and Special Supplemental Nutrition Program for Women, Infants and Children (WIC)

Guidelines for using stored breast milk for healthy, full-term babies.

BREAST MILK	ROOM 77°F (25°C) OR COLDER	REFRIGERATOR 40°F (4°C) OR COLDER	FREEZER SECTION 0°F (-18°C) OR COLDER
Fresh	Use within 4 hours	Use within 4 days	Use within 6 months
Thawed	Use within 2 hours	Use within 24 hours	Do not refreeze

These guidelines are for home use only and not for hospital use. If your baby is sick or premature, check with your baby's health care provider for storage recommendations.

Source: U.S. Department of Agriculture and Special Supplemental Nutrition Program for Women, Infants and Children (WIC)

Chapter 10

Eating for Two

Mothers have many questions concerning nutrition during breastfeeding.

How many calories should I eat while breast-feeding?

How can I lose the extra weight I gained during my pregnancy?

Are vitamin and mineral supplements necessary?

Though some health care providers recommend a strict diet for breastfeeding mothers, others suggest that mothers eat whatever they want. The following questions and answers can help you decide which foods are best for you and your baby.

Do I need to eat more calories?

Nutritional needs depend on how much milk is produced. For example, the woman who gives her baby formula in addition to breast milk does not need as many calories as the woman who breastfeeds twins. Milk production requires about 500 to 1,000 calories per day. Half of the calories come from body fat stored during pregnancy; the other half come from foods that you eat. Some nutritionists recommend that women eat 500 additional calories each day while breastfeeding. However, most women can produce enough milk while eating about the same number of calories as they did before they were pregnant. If

you want to lose the weight that you gained during pregnancy: Avoid high-calorie foods with no nutritional value; eat to satisfy your hunger; and try not to lose weight until your milk supply is well established—about 4–6 weeks after birth.

It is important to remember that the more you breastfeed, the more calories your body uses. The best weight loss is achieved when you breastfeed exclusively or almost exclusively for 6 months.

How can I lose the extra weight I gained during my pregnancy?

Most women find that they lose the extra weight gained during pregnancy over a 6-month period. Though this may seem like a long time, restricting calories to lose weight more quickly is not recommended since it can interfere with milk production. Although even malnourished mothers can produce high-quality milk, production is often at the expense of a mother's own health. By eating enough calories, you help ensure that your need for other nutrients, such as protein, vitamins, and minerals, is met as well.

If you were overweight before your pregnancy

Breastfeeding can help you lose weight. Once your milk supply is stable, eating 1,800 calories a day will maintain your milk supply and allow you to lose weight. If you do aerobic exercise or are very tall, you may need 2,000–2,400 calories a day. Your best guide is how fast you lose weight. Women who are obese should not lose more than 4–6 pounds a month. Women who need to lose 25 pounds or less should not lose more than 3–4 pounds a month.

If you were the right weight for your height before your pregnancy

Eating to satisfy your hunger and breastfeeding exclusively for about 6 months will result in a gradual return to your pre-pregnancy weight. As your baby reaches 6 months of age, you may find that you need to add calories to your diet to keep from losing too much weight. Remember that the minimum number of calories recommended is 1,800 each day. Again, women who are physically active or very tall may need 2,000–2,400 calories.

If you were underweight before your pregnancy

You may need to add some calories above your usual intake in order to keep from losing too much weight. This is especially important as your baby gets older, if you are exclusively breastfeeding. Weighing less than you did before your pregnancy should be avoided.

Do I need to drink extra fluid?

Your thirst is the best signal of how much fluid you should drink. In fact, excess fluids can actually decrease milk production. So follow

As long as you eat a balanced diet that includes a variety of foods, the only supplement you may need to take while breastfeeding is iron.

your own thirst (about six to eight servings of fluids a day) and drink healthy beverages such as water, low-fat or nonfat milk, and 100 percent fruit or vegetable juice. You can be sure you are getting enough to drink if your urine is clear or pale yellow.

Do I need to take vitamin and mineral supplements?

As long as you eat a balanced diet that includes a variety of foods, the only supplement you may need to take while breastfeeding is iron. Even if you do not menstruate (bleed each month) while exclusively breastfeeding, extra iron helps to replace the iron used during pregnancy.

If you have iron deficiency or iron deficiency anemia, your doctor will prescribe an iron supplement (60–120 mg a day). Remember that iron supplements are best absorbed on an empty stomach and should not be taken at the same time you take other nutrient supplements.

Some women avoid dairy products because of lactose intolerance, milk protein allergy, dislike of dairy products, or a vegan diet (strict vegetarian diet that does not include milk products). *If you do not eat dairy products or other high-calcium foods each day,* you should take a calcium supplement (600 mg a day).

Fortified dairy products are a source of vitamin D. *If you avoid dairy products and get less than 30 minutes of sun exposure a week,* you should take a vitamin D supplement (600 IU a day). The ultraviolet rays of the sun (with some help from the liver and kidneys) change a substance in the skin into vitamin D. Sunscreen blocks ultraviolet rays, so if you depend on sunlight for your vitamin D, wait for 30 minutes outdoors before you apply sunscreen. If you are in the sun often, you can wait less than 30 minutes.

Women who do not eat animal protein (meat, fish, eggs, or milk products) must choose foods carefully to get enough calories, protein, and nutrients, especially vitamin B12, iron, vitamin D, and zinc. Protein and other nutrients can be obtained by eating soy products and a variety of seeds, nuts, grains, legumes, vegetables, and cereals.

Do I need to limit the amount of fat in my diet?

You can limit the amount of fat in your diet by eating reduced-fat and nonfat foods such as mayonnaise, cream cheese, salad dressings, and cheese. But be sure to get some fat in your diet. If you are eating the minimum number of calories (1,800 a day), your diet should include 60 grams of fat. This may seem like a lot, but it is not. Every animal product you eat except for nonfat dairy products has fat. Lean chicken provides 2–3 grams of fat per ounce of meat. Beef and pork have 5–8 grams of fat per ounce. Fish has 1–5 grams of fat. Depending on the choices you make, it is easy to get 6–48 grams of fat from two small servings (3 ounces each) of high-protein foods per day. Balance a higher-fat protein choice with a lower-fat protein choice at the next meal.

You can limit the amount of saturated fat (the type in animal products) in your diet by keeping your protein servings small (2–4 ounces) and using monounsaturated and polyunsaturated oils in cooking.

Good oils include olive, canola, corn, flaxseed, sesame, soybean, safflower, and walnut. Remember, oils have 5 grams of fat per teaspoon.

Also, read labels on products such as mayonnaise, margarine, sour cream, and processed foods to check their fat content.

How can I increase the fatty acid content of my milk?

While the total amount of fat and the types of fatty acids in human milk may vary from one mother to another, human milk contains all the fatty acids a healthy, full-term baby needs. Some fatty acids cannot be made in the body and must be obtained from food sources. These are the *essential* fatty acids.

Others, like the long-chain polyunsaturated fatty acids, are made in the body but are also available in foods. Two long-chain polyunsaturated fatty acids that play an important role in visual development and brain function are docosahexaenoic acid (DHA) and arachidonic acid (ARA).

To ensure that your milk contains adequate amounts of DHA and ARA, include fatty fish (salmon, canned tuna, sardines, herring, anchovies) and vegetable oils (olive, canola, corn, safflower) in your diet.

Do I need to limit the amount of fish in my diet?

Fish are a good source of high-quality protein and are low in saturated fat. But nearly all fish contain mercury. So think small! Large fish that feed on smaller fish (swordfish, king mackerel, tilefish, shark, and tuna) often have high levels of mercury and should be eaten no more than once a month.

Farm-raised fish (especially salmon) are usually fed ground-up fish that contain high levels of PCBs and other cancer-causing chemicals. Many producers of farm-raised fish are trying to improve the quality of the food that is fed to their fish. Many fish are now labeled, so it easier to tell if they are farm-raised or caught in the wild. Farm-raised fish should be eaten no more than once or twice a month.

You can still enjoy the health benefits of seafood by eating shellfish (shrimp, scallops, crab, squid, and lobster), canned fish (sardines, herring, and anchovies), or smaller ocean fish (wild salmon, cod, and sole).

Is it true that some foods can make my baby fussy?

Something in your diet may make your baby fussy now and then. Foods that sometimes cause fussiness include milk products, eggs, and nuts. If you have a family history of allergic disease or a very fussy baby, you might want to limit these foods in your diet.

Small amounts of caffeine (the equivalent of one or two cups of regular coffee a day) are considered safe for breastfeeding mothers and healthy, full-term babies. But large amounts of caffeine (the equivalent of five or more cups of regular coffee a day) can cause fussy, wakeful babies. If you have a fussy baby, you might want to limit your intake of caffeine-containing drinks and foods such as coffee, tea, chocolate, and some carbonated beverages (see table). The amount of caffeine in a cup of coffee or tea depends upon the brewing method and the ingredients.

Will certain foods change the color of my milk?

Certain foods or medicines can cause your milk to change color. The most common colors are orange, green, or black. If you notice a change in the color of your milk, make a list of the foods or medicines you have taken recently that might be the cause. If the color change persists, contact your doctor or your baby's doctor. As long as your baby shows no

Caffeine content of drinks and foods.

DRINK / FOOD	CAFFEINE
Drip coffee 7 oz	115–175 mg
Percolator coffee 7 oz	80–135 mg
Instant coffee 7 oz	65–100 mg
Brewed tea 7 oz	40–60 mg
Instant tea 7 oz	30 mg
Iced tea 12 oz	70 mg
Mountain Dew 12 oz	54 mg
Mello Yello 12 oz	53 mg
Coca-Cola 12 oz	46 mg
Diet Coke 12 oz	46 mg
Dr. Pepper 12 oz	40 mg
Pepsi-Cola 12 oz	38 mg
Diet Pepsi 12 oz	36 mg
Milk chocolate 1 oz	6 mg
Dark chocolate 1 oz	20 mg

signs of illness such as vomiting, diarrhea, or fever, you can continue to breastfeed.

Can I use artificial sweeteners?

Small amounts of artificial sweeteners such as saccharin and aspartame are thought to be safe. Saccharin is a weak cancer-causing substance. The safe level of daily intake is 500 mg for children and 1,000 mg for adults. A popular brand of artificial sweetener using saccharin has about 14–20 mg per packet.

Aspartame causes an increase in the level of phenylalanine and should not be used by individuals with phenylketonuria (PKU). There's no proof that aspartame harms breastfed babies, but moderate use (no more than two to four servings a day) of artificial sweeteners and artificially sweetened beverages is recommended.

Can I drink alcohol?

Drinking small amounts of alcohol (4 ounces of wine, 12 ounces of beer, or 1 ounce of spirits such as whiskey, rum, vodka, or gin) no more than once a week is thought to be safe. However, alcohol can change the flavor of your milk, shorten your breastfeeding sessions, decrease your milk supply, and limit your baby's weight gain. Daily use of alcohol, even in small amounts, can affect your baby's motor development (e.g., ability to crawl, walk, grasp, hold) and your ability to care for your baby. To limit the effects of alcohol on you and your baby, drink no more than one or two drinks a week and try not to breastfeed for at least 2 hours after you drink.

Can I smoke?

Smoking affects the breastfeeding mother and baby in many ways. It lowers the nutritional status of the mother, decreases the metabolism of vitamin B12, alters zinc bal-ance in the body, and lowers the levels of vitamin C and folic acid. Smoking causes a decrease in prolactin and oxytocin, a decrease in the fat content of milk, and a decrease in milk production, which can lead to early weaning. Because the many benefits of breastfeeding outweigh the risks of smoking, mothers who smoke are still encouraged to breastfeed. However, to limit the effects of second-hand smoke on your baby, reduce the number of cigarettes you smoke to no more than five a day, and do not smoke in the house, in the car, or near your baby.

How can I improve my diet to produce the highest quality milk possible?

- Eat the recommended number of servings (see table on next page).

- Eat a fish meal (especially cold water fish like wild salmon) two or three times a week. If you eat fish that contain high levels of mercury (like swordfish) limit your intake to no more than once a month.

- Use nonfat milk products and a variety of oils.

- Eat a minimum of 1,800 calories a day.

- Select foods that provide important nutrients (see table on next page).

Suggested breastfeeding diet.

FOOD GROUP	NUMBER OF SERVINGS	EXAMPLES OF ONE SERVING	
WHOLE-GRAIN BREAD, CEREAL, RICE, PASTA	6–11	1	slice bread
		½	roll, muffin, biscuit
		1	tortilla
		½ cup	hot cereal
		1 cup	ready-to-eat cereal
		½ cup	rice, noodles, pasta
FRUIT	2–4	¾ cup	fruit juice
		1	orange, apple, banana, pear
		½	grapefruit
		½ cup	chopped, cooked, or canned fruit
		½ cup	berries
		1 slice	melon
		¼ cup	dried fruit
VEGETABLES	3–5	¾ cup	vegetable juice
		½ cup	cooked vegetables like broccoli, green beans, peas, turnip greens, kale
		½ cup	chopped raw vegetables
		1 cup	raw leafy vegetables like spinach, lettuce, endive
MEAT, POULTRY, FISH, DRY BEANS/PEAS, EGGS, NUTS	3	2–3 oz	lean meat, fish, poultry
		1	egg
		½ cup	cooked beans
		2 tbsp	peanut butter
		½ cup	canned tuna
		½ cup	tofu
		2½ oz	soy burger
		⅓ cup	nuts or seeds
MILK, MILK PRODUCTS	3–4	1 cup	milk
		1 cup	yogurt
		1½ cup	cottage cheese
		1½ oz	natural cheese
		2 oz	processed cheese like American
		1½ cups	ice cream
FATS, OILS	Small amounts	1 tsp	butter, mayonnaise, oil
		1 tbsp	salad dressing
		1 tbsp	sour cream

Foods containing important nutrients.

FOLIC ACID	CALCIUM	ZINC
leafy vegetables	milk	beef
green beans	yogurt	poultry
legumes	cheese	seafood
fortified cereals	sardines/salmon with bones	eggs
fruit	dark green leafy vegetables	pork
	dried beans and peas	fortified cereals
	fortified orange juice	yogurt
	fortified tofu	legumes
	fortified tortillas	seeds

VITAMIN A	VITAMIN B	VITAMIN C
dark green leafy vegetables	banana	citrus fruits and juices
orange/yellow vegetables	watermelon	fortified juices
liver	meat	strawberries
egg yolk	potatoes	broccoli
cheese	sweet potatoes	cabbage
milk	nuts/seeds	potatoes
butter	fortified cereals	green peppers

Chapter 11

Breastfeeding and Working

Many mothers who work outside the home continue to breastfeed. It takes a little extra planning, but the benefits are worth it. See Chapter 2, "Benefits of Breastfeeding."

- Breastfeeding keeps a mother and baby close even when they are apart.

- Breast milk keeps babies healthy (especially those in group child care centers).

- Mothers of healthy babies miss less work, lose less income, and worry less about sick babies.

- Breastfeeding saves money; mothers who breastfeed do not have to buy large amounts of infant formula or foods to replace their breast milk.

Many mothers don't realize that combining breastfeeding and working is possible, so they stop breastfeeding when they return to work. But as the number of working mothers increases, employers are becoming more supportive of breastfeeding. In the past, few employers considered breastfeeding beneficial, but today many see how breastfeeding can help their business.

Key points to think about

As you plan how you will combine breastfeeding and working, here are some key points to think about:

- How do you plan to feed your baby when you return to work?

- How will you express your milk or feed your baby during working hours?

- How will you complete your work duties and take care of your breastfeeding needs?

- How will you combine work duties and household chores?

Start planning before your baby is born

Let your employer know as soon as possible that you are pregnant. Use this time to learn about your company's maternity policies, benefits, and work options. Discuss these options with your employer; suggest new options if necessary.

- How long is your maternity leave? Is it paid or unpaid? How much leave can you take without losing your job or position? Does your national, state, or local government have a family medical leave law? (Some laws provide up to 12 weeks of unpaid maternity leave.)

- How many hours per week will you be expected to work when you return?

- Does your employer offer work options such as flex-time (adjusting when you start and

Second trimester
Meet with your employer.

stop work each day), job-sharing (sharing a full-time job with another person), part-time work, compressed work week (fewer days with longer hours), or telecommuting (working from home)?

- Do your employer's policies allow you to leave the work site during the day or have an infant at work part or full time?

- Does your employer offer on-site child care? If not, is this an option your employer might consider?

- Does your employer have a policy on breast-feeding or milk expression at the work site? Does your employer provide breast pumps or breastfeeding rooms? Does your employer give employees time and support to breastfeed or express milk during the work day? (This is very important.)

Decide when you will return to work

Once you know the policies of your company, you can think about your options.

The longer you and your baby can be together, the more stable your milk supply will be. Also, the older your baby is when you return to work, the less you may need to pump during the work day.

It is best to take off as much time as possible. Whether you return to work after 6 weeks, 6 months, or 6 years will depend on your own needs and circumstances. For many mothers, the decision to return to work is not a choice but a necessity. Mothers with limited sources of income and no paid maternity leave have to return to paid work as soon as possible.

Third trimester
Attend a prenatal
breastfeeding class.

Decide how many hours a week you would like to work and when

Mothers who are able to work part time at first will find it easier to work and breastfeed. A part-time schedule gives you a chance to rest and care for yourself and your baby, and makes the return to work easier. Mothers who return to work full time right away are sometimes able to work flexible hours that allow extra time during the work day for expressing their milk or breastfeeding. Others compress their work week, completing a full-time schedule in fewer than 5 days—for example, working a 40-hour week in four 10-hour days or three 13-hour days.

Many mothers successfully combine breastfeeding and working. You simply need to plan ahead.

Decide where and when you can express or breastfeed at work

If you plan to return to work shortly after your baby is born and want to express or breastfeed at the work site, think about where and when this can happen. You won't know how long breastfeeding or expressing your milk will take until after your baby is born and you have had a chance to practice, but you can plan ahead. Look for places at the work site where you can express your milk or breastfeed, such as a private office, a health clinic, or a child care center. You may need to be creative as you look for space, privacy, and comfort.

If you plan to use a breast pump, find out if your employer provides a pump and supplies, or ask for these as a baby gift.

Decide who will take care of your baby while you are at work

Choosing child care is an important task. While cost and convenience are necessary considerations, choosing someone you trust who understands and supports breastfeeding is very important.

Child care options include taking your baby to work with you; leaving your baby with an individual, in either your home or theirs; taking your baby to a child care center; or arranging work schedules so that one parent is always available to care for your baby.

If you plan to breastfeed your baby during working hours, you might want to choose an individual or child care center near your work place or arrange to have your baby brought to you for feedings.

When you are interviewing different child care providers, ask them about their policies concerning breastfed babies. Choose someone who understands and supports breastfeeding and who is licensed or certified (especially if you are considering a group child care center). Take plenty of time to interview possible providers, and make at least one unscheduled visit.

You need to know that your baby will get the care you want. Choose a provider who:

- provides a safe, clean place for your baby.

- encourages you to breastfeed on-site when you drop off or pick up your baby, as well as during the day.

- has an adequate number of trained staff who have experience in infant care and will help meet your baby's special needs.

- is near your work site, if you are able to leave work to feed your baby.

- knows how to safely handle your expressed breast milk and feed your baby.

If you have a child care center at your work site, let your employer know how much you value this employee benefit. If you do not have on-site child care, get information from other companies who provide this service and share the information with your employer.

Get support from your employer, supervisor, and co-workers

Before you begin your maternity leave, discuss your ideas with your supervisor and co-workers. Encourage them to support your efforts to breastfeed after you return to work. See if you can get them to commit their support in writing.

Some ideas for building and maintaining support with your employer include:

- Talking with other working, breastfeeding mothers about their situations at their workplaces. If they have had positive experiences, see if their supervisors would be willing to discuss the arrangement(s) with your employer. Sometimes employers are more willing to follow where others have already shown success, rather than being the first to offer special services.

- Sharing research data or publications on how breastfeeding can help businesses. For instance, breastfed babies are typically sick fewer times, even when placed in group day care centers. Less sickness on your baby's part means less absence on your part, which means better productivity for the company. According to one study, nonbreastfeeding mothers were absent from their jobs three times more often (due to babies' illnesses) than breastfeeding mothers.

- Exploring ways to meet your job responsibilities while you are breastfeeding, so that your employer, supervisor, and co-workers will agree that you are doing your fair share of the work.

Breastfeed early and often

Enjoy this precious time with your baby to the fullest. Breastfeed early and often. This will help your baby learn good breastfeeding practices and help you establish a good milk supply. Avoid pacifiers, bottles, or foods other than breast milk for the first 4 weeks after birth. These can confuse your baby and decrease your milk supply.

Learn how to express your milk

You will need to learn to express breast milk if you plan to have your milk given to your baby during the workday.

Once your baby is born you can begin to practice hand expression. You can also begin to use a simple hand pump, a battery-operated pump, or an electric pump (see "Choosing a Breast Pump," page 66).

Practice early and often so that you will have time to learn this important skill before you return to work.

Your first attempts at milk expression may produce only enough milk to cover the bottom of the collection container. Don't get discouraged. Much like successful breastfeeding, successful milk expression comes with practice. See Chapter 9, "Expressing and Storing Your Milk."

Birth	Breastfeed as soon as possible.
1–2 weeks	Breastfeed at least eight times in each 24 hours.
2–4 weeks	Learn to express and collect your milk; freeze milk for later use.
4–10 weeks	Introduce a bottle or cup.
6–12 weeks	Delay your return to work for 12 weeks if possible.

After you have expressed your milk, you can store it in just about any food storage container. There are even plastic bags made just for breast milk. Use something that is not likely to break, tear, or tip over in the refrigerator or freezer.

If you are expressing early on, and your baby is breastfeeding well, freeze your milk for later use. Label it with the date it was expressed.

Breast milk can be stored in a cool room for up to 4 hours, in the refrigerator for up to 4 days, and in the freezer for up to 6 months (or longer).

As your baby gets older and your return to work gets closer, store your milk in single servings. Of course, your baby may want a bit more or less than this amount on any given day. If your baby seems hungrier than usual, feel free to make up larger servings for your baby's child care provider, or send along extra servings. Remember to adjust serving size as your baby grows.

Estimate the size of a single serving

During the first 1–6 months, healthy, full-term babies drink about 25 ounces (750 ml) of breast milk each day. Some babies drink as little as 19 ounces a day (570 ml) while others drink as much as 30 ounces a day (900 ml). You can estimate the size of a single serving by dividing 25 ounces by the number of daily breastfeedings. For example, if your baby breastfeeds eight times a day, divide 25 by 8 and you will find that your baby needs about 3 ounces per feeding when you are away.

Introduce a new feeding method and/or breast milk substitute

Once your baby is breastfeeding well, about 4 weeks after birth, you can introduce a new feeding method. If you do this too soon, you can confuse your baby. However, if your work schedule requires that you be away from your baby during feeding times, you need to know that she will accept food from something other than the breast and from someone other than you.

What to substitute

Depending on your baby's age and ability, you can use expressed breast milk, infant formula, or solid food. Doctors recommend breast milk alone for about the first 6 months.

If you cannot provide breast milk, your baby's doctor can recommend an infant formula.

After the first 6 months, solid foods can be introduced, but breast milk or infant formula should still be an important part of your baby's diet for at least the first year.

How to substitute

You can use a spoon, cup, medicine dropper, hollow-handled medicine spoon, or bottle—whichever you, your baby, and your child care provider prefer.

Should you choose to place the substitute in a bottle, try different nipple shapes and sizes until you find one that your baby will accept.

Let someone other than you offer the substitute—your baby expects meals from you to come from your breast, not a cup or a bottle! You may want to leave the room during the feeding, since some babies refuse substitutes when the real thing is nearby. Your partner or your baby's grandmother, babysitter, brother, or sister may be more than happy to offer the feeding.

You can avoid substitutes by letting your baby sleep during the day while you are at work and breastfeed in the evening and at night when you are together. This works well if you don't mind the interrupted sleep.

Decide how to combine household chores and work duties

When both parents work full time outside the home, household chores are often shared. While cooking, cleaning, doing laundry, paying bills, grocery shopping, and running errands take time and energy, now breastfeeding and child care must be added to the to-do list!

- Sit down with your partner and make a list of all your household chores.

- Decide which chores can be put off, and divide up the rest.

Return to work

During your pregnancy and maternity leave, you laid out your plans. Now that you and your baby have learned to breastfeed, it's time to put these plans into action.

Two weeks before your scheduled return to work

- Discuss your plans with your supervisor. Assure her/him that you will be able to maintain your agreed-upon daily and weekly work schedule.

- See how much time you will need each workday to wake, dress, feed yourself and your baby, and travel to child care and work.

- Let your babysitter and baby spend time together, so they get to know one another.

- Begin to establish a milk expression schedule, if you will be expressing milk at work.

- If you will not be able to express milk at work, drop one feeding during the day and introduce a substitute, so that your milk supply has a chance to adjust. If you need to drop a second daily feeding, wait 3–5 days.

- Introduce a substitute to your baby at the time you would otherwise breastfeed.

- Start making extra meals for you and your partner and storing them in the freezer.

2 weeks before you return to work
Decide how much time you will need each
workday to get yourself and your baby ready.

1 week before you return to work
Hold a dress rehearsal.

After you return to work
Make the most of your time together.

One week before your scheduled return to work

- Continue your expression and breastfeeding schedule so that it will be close to what you will be doing when you return to work.

- Leave your baby with your child care provider for a few hours two or three times this week so they can get to know one another.

- Hold a dress rehearsal of your new morning routine on 1 or 2 days this week, and make changes as needed.

- Try to get plenty of sleep so that you are ready for your return to work.

When you return to work

- Take one day at a time. If work has piled up while you were away, relax and do your best to catch up.

- If you return to work full time, try to work only 2 or 3 days the first week. For example, if your work week occurs Monday through Friday, return to work on a Wednesday or Thursday.

- Breastfeed your baby right before you leave her with your child care provider. This will limit the amount of milk you will need to express while you are apart.

- Express or breastfeed according to your established routine. You will probably need to make small adjustments depending on your work schedule. Try to express or breastfeed a little early rather than a little late. Many times the hours rush by and you may find yourself having gone longer than planned. If you do not express or breastfeed, milk is more likely to leak from your breasts, you will feel uncomfortably full, and your milk supply may decrease.

- Breastfeed your baby right after you return from work. If your breasts are very full or you have a long commute home, you may want to breastfeed before you leave the child care center. This will keep you and your baby happy. Ask your child care provider not to feed your baby for 1–2 hours before your planned return, so that she will be ready to eat when you get there.

- Breastfeed more often in the evenings and on weekends when you and your baby are together. This will help to maintain your milk supply.

- Talk with your supervisor about how things are going. Be positive and thankful, but also be open and honest if there are difficulties.

- Take care of yourself. Commit to getting enough sleep and eating a healthy diet.

- If you notice a decrease in your milk supply, don't panic! Once you adjust to your new routine, your milk supply should return to normal. In the meantime, try to squeeze in an extra pumping session when you are at work or some extra breastfeedings when you and your baby are together.

- Give your baby at least one substitute feeding each day during any days off work (weekends, vacations, holidays).

Regardless of how well you prepare for your return to work, there will still be a period of adjustment. Excitement, nervousness, guilt, sadness, and joy are a few of the emotions you may experience. These feelings are normal. With time you will adjust priorities and establish routines, and your confidence in your decision will grow. Support and encouragement from people around you are important, so don't hesitate to ask for help.

Any amount of breastfeeding is wonderful. More important than how long you breastfeed or how often is that it be enjoyable for you and your baby.

Combining breast pumping and working will help you maintain your milk supply.

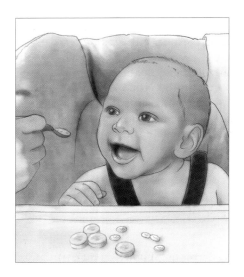

Chapter 12

Weaning Your Baby

Any amount of breastfeeding is good for you and your baby. Some mothers breastfeed for several weeks, some for several months, and others for several years. How long you breastfeed depends on your own needs and the needs of your child.

Breast milk provides all the nutrients your baby needs for the first 6 months of life. Even after solid foods are introduced, breast milk should still be an important part of your baby's diet for at least the first year.

Social or cultural pressures cause some mothers to wean. Others wean because of the demands of work or school. Sometimes the separation of mother and baby health reasons makes weaning necessary. More important than when you wean or why is that you wean slowly.

In many Western cultures, where independence is valued, a baby's first tooth or first step can be seen as a sign that it is time to wean. In reality, the right time to wean is when your child, your partner, or you decide that the time is right. Though family and friends may be eager to offer advice about why, when, and how to wean, only you know what is best for you and your child.

Even small amounts of breast milk are valuable. The longer a mother and child breastfeed, the greater the benefits for both. The American Academy of Pediatrics, the World Health Organization, and the United Nations Children's Fund (UNICEF) all recommend exclusive breastfeeding for the first 6 months of life, and continued breastfeeding along with complementary foods for at least 1–2 years.

Despite these recommendations, women in Western cultures who choose to breastfeed beyond the first year often face the disapproval of family and friends.

Fortunately, cultures change, albeit slowly. In the meantime, surround yourself with people who support your decision to breastfeed, whether it be for 1, 2, or more years!

When should I start my baby on solid foods?

There is no magical age at which all babies are suddenly ready for solid foods. Babies grow and develop at their own pace, so it is important to watch your baby for signs indicating that he is ready for solid foods. These signs include the ability to:

- sit up without support

- control his head

- bring food to his mouth

- swallow solid foods without choking

 Moms and dads share tips on how to know your baby is ready for solid foods:

babygooroo.com/video/solids

Most babies show an interest in solid foods around 6 months of age and delight in taking food from nearby plates. These early solid food feedings are a learning experience for you and your baby. So don't be surprised to find that most of the food ends up everywhere except your baby's mouth!

How do I begin weaning?

Weaning is a gradual process of babies "taking hold" and mothers "letting go." Weaning begins naturally when solid food or liquids other than breast milk are introduced, and it continues until breast milk has been completely replaced by other foods.

The weaning process can last for days, weeks, months, or years. Mothers in Western cultures tend to wean earlier than mothers in non-Western cultures, although weaning at a later age is becoming more common. The average age for weaning worldwide is 2–4 years, and in some cultures children breastfeed for 5–7 years—the breast is a wonderful place to eat, sleep, and cuddle!

Weaning is easiest when both mother and child are ready and willing, but more often one or the other leads the way. Given enough time, nearly all children will wean themselves, but culture plays an important role in the decision to wean. Many mothers in Western cultures, where extended breastfeeding is less common, are reluctant to breastfeed beyond the toddler years.

More important than when you wean or why is that the process be gradual. Weaning, particularly if it is sudden, may cause mothers to feel sad or guilty. These feelings are made worse if the baby is unwilling to stop breastfeeding. Feelings of sadness may be due in part to the decrease in prolactin but are more likely due to the unexpected end of the breastfeeding relationship.

Some mothers are ready to give up the closeness that breastfeeding provides while others are not. Most mothers have mixed feelings about weaning. These feelings are common and will pass with time, but it may help to talk openly and honestly about your feelings with people you trust.

You may also find it helpful to remember that the benefits of breastfeeding continue long after breastfeeding stops.

Suggestions for weaning slowly

- Replace one daily breastfeeding at a time with solids or liquids, depending on your baby's age and ability. Choose the breastfeedings in which your baby is the least interested.

- If your baby is under 1 year of age, use iron-fortified formula for replacement feedings. Cow's milk should be avoided until your baby is at least 1 year old, and then be sure to use whole and not low-fat milk.

- Once your baby can sit up, control his head, and bring food to his mouth, he is ready for solid foods. This usually happens at about 6 months of age. Giving solid foods for the first time can be an adventure, so get ready!

- Choose foods that will meet your baby's need for iron. Meats and iron-fortified cereals are suggested.

- Wait 5–7 days before you offer each new food, so that you can watch for signs of allergy.

- Place liquids in a bottle or a cup depending on your baby's age and ability. Even newborns can learn to cup-feed, so you may

prefer to use a cup and avoid bottles and nipples altogether. If you use a bottle, try different nipple shapes until you find one your baby will accept. A slow-flow nipple may lessen the difference between bottle-feeding and breastfeeding. If you use a cup and your baby is able to sit up and hold the cup by himself, you might want to use a cup with two handles and a snap-on lid to prevent spills.

- Often babies refuse foods offered by their mother, so you may need to ask another family member to help with replacement

Once your baby can sit up, control his head, and bring food to his mouth, he is ready for solid foods.

feedings. After many months of breast-feeding, partners, brothers, and sisters are usually eager for a chance to feed the baby.

- Replace one daily breastfeeding no sooner than every 3–5 days until weaning is complete. Many babies are reluctant to give up the early morning, naptime, and bedtime feedings. If your baby resists, you can continue to breastfeed at those times, but try to shorten the length of feedings.

- Increase cuddling time. Your baby needs to know that separation from the breast does not mean separation from you. Hugs and kisses will let your baby know that your love and affection continue even after breast-feeding stops.

- Distract an active and curious toddler with games, outdoor play, and story-telling.

- Offer soft finger foods that appeal to young children, such as banana, scrambled egg, cooked peas, and iron-fortified cereal.

- Expect some breast milk production to continue for many days or even many weeks after weaning is complete.

Suggestions for sudden weaning

- Hand express or pump to relieve fullness. A warm washcloth or a warm shower or bath can make milk expression easier. Remove only enough milk to relieve fullness and prevent engorgement. The more milk you remove from your breasts, the more milk you will make.

- Put ice on your breasts to relieve pain and reduce swelling. Cold packs, bags of frozen peas wrapped in wet washcloths, or cold, rinsed cabbage leaves work well (see page 105).

- If necessary, ask your health care provider to recommend a pain-relieving medication.

- Wear a snug bra for comfort and support.

Chapter 13

Breastfeeding Beyond the First Year

Breastfeeding isn't just for babies! Many mothers and toddlers cherish the special relationship that breastfeeding provides and continue to breastfeed beyond the first year. Most health professional organizations recommend that children be breastfed for 2 years or more.

Depending on your child's needs, you can continue to breastfeed for 2, 3, or more years. Breastfeeding an older baby or toddler can be rewarding as well as challenging.

Do the benefits of breastfeeding continue beyond the first year?

The benefits of breastfeeding continue as long as you continue to breastfeed. Although the emotional benefits of breastfeeding are most often given as the reason for breastfeeding an older baby or toddler, breastfed babies of all ages enjoy better health. Other foods provide toddlers with important nutrients, but only breast milk contains antibodies that play a role in preventing disease.

Here are just a few of the benefits of breastfeeding beyond the first year:

- Breast milk can provide toddlers with up to a third of their calorie, protein, and calcium needs.

- Breast milk continues to create antibodies that fight infection and illness during the second year and beyond.

- If a breastfed toddler does get sick, the illness often lasts for a shorter period of time.

- If a sick toddler refuses to eat, breast milk may be the only source of nourishment that she will accept.

- Studies suggest that breastfeeding for a longer period of time may result in even smarter babies.

Mothers also benefit from breastfeeding beyond the first year:

- Women who breastfeed exclusively for the first 6 months are less likely to get pregnant, so child spacing is easier.

- The longer a mother breastfeeds, the less risk she has of breast, ovarian, and uterine cancer.

- Women with diabetes find that their insulin needs continue to be lower while they are breastfeeding.

For older babies who prefer to "eat and run," breastfeeding offers a quick and easy snack. Breastfeeding also provides help in falling asleep, comfort after getting hurt, and reassurance when mothers and babies are reunited after a separation. Because breastfeeding is something that only mothers can do for their babies, many busy mothers, especially those returning to work or school, find that breastfeeding makes it easier for them to reconnect with their babies at the end of the day.

Years later, a mother who breastfed her toddler can still recall his tiny hands gently patting or rubbing her face during breastfeeding. She remembers the special love she felt as her baby looked into her eyes and smiled, still attached to her breast. She can also recall the sweet baby sounds and simple words that told her how special breastfeeding was to her baby.

Is breastfeeding a toddler different from breastfeeding an infant?

Breastfeeding a toddler is very different from breastfeeding an infant. Most breastfeedings are short and sweet, but the frequency can vary from once every other day to several times each day. Because toddlers eat a wide variety of foods, they don't need to breastfeed at certain times. If a mother and baby are out and about during the usual feeding time, the older baby will usually accept some other food or drink without a fuss. Some toddlers will insist on breastfeeding, regardless of the time and place. As they get older, they will be more willing to wait.

Breastfeeding an older baby can be an adventure. Toddlers are very aware of what's going on around them. Don't be surprised if your toddler lets go of the breast to watch the cat, smile at dad, or simply react to a noise. You might think this means that your baby is losing interest in breastfeeding. However, this behavior is normal and is one of the ways babies learn. Some toddlers turn away from the breast but don't let go, testing the ability of the breast to stretch! This doesn't mean that breastfeeding must stop. But because some toddlers are so easily distracted, you may need to breastfeed your toddler in a quiet place.

As babies get older, sleeping patterns change, too. Some breastfed babies sleep for long periods of time right from the start, and by 1 or 2 years of age are sleeping all night. Others continue to wake at night to breastfeed, especially if they are not offered regular meals and snacks during the day. Parents' habits also affect the older baby's sleeping schedule. If you are a night owl, your toddler may be one also.

What will my friends and family think?

Everyone has opinions about how you should raise your baby. And, unfortunately, most are eager to share their opinions, which often include feelings about how long you should breastfeed. You and your partner will have to decide what is best for you and your baby and ignore advice that is not supportive.

Family members may frown on long-term breastfeeding. They may believe that breast milk provides no nutrition or benefits after the first year. The whole idea of breastfeeding a baby that looks like a child may make them feel uncomfortable. And they may make it their mission to convince you to change your mind about continuing to breastfeed.

Be prepared to deal with family members' questions and comments. Share the facts about breastfeeding to win their support when possible. If you are asked repeatedly to say how long you intend to breastfeed, you can truthfully say that you have started weaning. Weaning actually does begin when your baby starts to eat foods other than breast milk. However, the end of breastfeeding may not happen for many months or years.

Many people believe that breastfeeding beyond a certain age will make children too dependent or "tied" to mom. But research suggests that just the opposite is true. Children who form a secure attachment with their mother are better able to form relationships with others and are more likely to be independent.

Negative comments from family and friends are seldom meant to be hurtful. Your family and friends care about you and your child and want what is best for you, even if their information is wrong. Find out their specific concerns so that you will know how to respond. Tell them what the doctor or other expert has said about breastfeeding an older child.

Overall, most parents find that their family and friends quickly get used to the idea of breastfeeding an older baby. Many women who breastfed a year or more say that at first they couldn't picture themselves breastfeeding a toddler. But over time, breast-feeding a walking, talking toddler began to feel natural and normal.

What challenges will I face breastfeeding an older baby?

Breastfeeding in public

Many mothers continue to breastfeed beyond the first year but do so only in a private place or in their home. Most people accept the need to breastfeed a young infant whenever and wherever she gets hungry. They usually smile with approval or just look away. However, they may not feel the same about older babies breastfeeding. A common belief is that a mother who breastfeeds an older baby is doing so for her own satisfaction. Some mothers have experienced rude comments or stares, or have been asked to leave a place. For some people, seeing an older baby breast-feeding stirs up feelings of anger or disgust.

There are many ways to handle questions, comments, or looks that may make you feel uncomfortable. First, draw as little attention as possible by covering up with a shawl, scarf, or child's blanket. Second, ask a family member or friend to hold your baby or toddler so that she doesn't ask to breastfeed in public by pulling at your blouse or breast. Third, teach your toddler to use a code word for breastfeeding that does not suggest that you may still be breastfeeding. Most toddlers will ask to breastfeed even if the mother has never done so in public. Toddlers can wait to breastfeed and can eat other foods, so you may find it easier to just avoid breastfeeding in public.

If you choose to breastfeed in public, know that by doing so, you can give other mothers the confidence they need to do the same. As breastfeeding becomes more common, women will care more about the needs of their children and less about the opinions of others.

Breastfeeding and biting

Babies often have six to eight teeth by 1 year of age, but fortunately, it's impossible for babies to bite and breastfeed at the same time. When a baby is latched on well, the mother's nipple extends far back into the baby's mouth. The nipple does not come into contact with the baby's teeth. Not all babies bite, and biting does not have to end breastfeeding.

Biting tends to occur near the end of a feeding when a baby is full or when a baby really isn't hungry. You can reduce the chances that your baby will bite by watching for signs that your baby has finished feeding and removing him from the breast.

Biting can also occur while a mother is talking on the phone or not interacting with her baby. Give your baby your full attention while breastfeeding, and breastfeed in a quiet place.

Sometimes biting issues begin early if a baby is allowed to bite or pinch a mother's arm, neck, or face during play. A baby does not know that biting the breast is different, so do not allow playful biting involving your-self or anyone else. Babies find comfort in rubbing their gums against something when their gums are sore during teething. Try rubbing your baby's gums with your fingers and use a chilled, firm teething ring to soothe his gums between breastfeedings.

If your baby does bite, avoid smiling, laughing, or reacting in a way that makes your baby think it was funny or cute. Calmly press your baby's face into your breast. This causes your baby to release your nipple. Then remove your baby from the breast and firmly say "no." Toddlers are able to understand your dislike for their behavior. Wait until the next usual feeding time to allow your baby to breastfeed again. Biting may occur only once if dealt with quickly. Like other stages in your baby's life, biting will become a thing of the past.

Will breastfeeding cause my toddler not to eat or grow well?

Breastfeeding toddlers will usually accept solid foods as long as the foods are introduced between 6 and 12 months of age. That seems to be the time when babies are ready to explore a variety of flavors and textures.

Moms share tips on breastfeeding a baby who has teeth:

babygooroo.com/video/biting

Regular meals and snacks plus continued breastfeeding will help to keep your older baby healthy.

Some parents put off adding foods because they think foods are not needed until after 1 year of age if the baby is breastfeeding. When parents delay giving foods at the age when babies are ready, eating may become a battle. As a result, the toddler may not grow as well as expected. Toddlers who refuse to eat or who eat very little may have been allowed to breastfeed too frequently in place of eating solid foods.

Parents may put off adding chunky or table foods until after 1 year because they are worried about choking. While it is a good idea to avoid some foods like hot dogs, grapes, or nuts, most soft foods are safe for toddlers. If toddlers have been given only smooth or pureed foods, they may fear foods with texture and refuse to eat. But if foods with texture and shape are added gradually, the baby will learn to handle the foods without a problem.

Where can I find support in my community for breastfeeding an older child?

Mothers who are breastfeeding toddlers often find strength in numbers. Many communities offer mother-to-mother support groups such as those sponsored by La Leche League International. For more information on the resources in your area, contact your health care provider or your baby's health care provider.

How long you and your baby decide to breastfeed is a decision only you and your baby can make, so don't let the opinions of others influence you.

Many mothers and toddlers cherish the special relationship that breastfeeding provides.

WHAT-IF'S

Chapter 14

Managing Possible Problems

The more you learn about how to breastfeed, the less likely you are to have problems while breastfeeding. It is best to prevent problems before they occur. But problems can happen despite your best efforts. If you know what signs to look for, you can pick up on problems early and start treatment right away.

Breast engorgement

Signs

Nearly all women experience breast fullness during the first 2–3 days after their babies are born. Do not confuse normal fullness with engorgement. Engorged breasts are swollen, hard, and painful, and your skin is red, shiny, and hot. Your body temperature can increase slightly (to less than 100°F or 37.7°C).

Cause

After your baby is born, your blood carries fluid and nutrients to your breasts so that you can make enough milk to meet your baby's needs. This added fluid causes your breasts to swell. Frequent breastfeedings or milk expression will reduce the swelling and soften your breasts. If breastfeedings are infrequent, delayed, or missed, your breasts overfill and fluid collects, causing engorgement.

Recommended treatment

- Put cold packs on your breasts to reduce the swelling. Bags of frozen peas wrapped in a wet washcloth work well. Some women use cold, raw cabbage leaves on their breasts after each feeding to reduce engorgement. Why cabbage leaves relieve engorgement is unclear. There may be a substance in the leaves that reduces swelling, or it may be the cool temperature of the leaves. Rinse the leaves in cold water before use. Place the leaves on your breasts with your nipples exposed until the leaves wilt. Apply fresh leaves only until the swelling decreases.

- Hand express or pump a small amount of milk. This will soften your breasts and make it easier for your baby to latch on correctly (see "Hand Expressing," page 64). Taking a warm shower or bath may make milk expression easier. Heat, however, can also increase swelling, so do not use heat unless your breasts are leaking freely.

- Breastfeed frequently during the day and at night. To increase the flow of milk, gently massage your breast in a circular pattern while your baby is breastfeeding, using the flat part of your fingers. If your breasts are still full and firm after feeding, hand express or pump to relieve fullness.

- Wear a bra for comfort and support. Avoid bras that are too tight or that bind, making it difficult to relieve fullness and soften your breasts. Avoid bras with underwires. If you prefer a bra with underwires, remove the bra for one or two feedings during the day and at night.

To prevent engorgement

- Breastfeed as soon as possible after birth.

- Breastfeed frequently during the day and at night. Do not skip nighttime feedings.

- Breastfeed as long as your baby wishes on the first breast before offering the second breast. If necessary, hand express or pump to relieve fullness in the second breast.

- Offer both breasts at every feeding.

- Begin each feeding on the breast offered last.

- If you delay or miss a feeding or your baby breastfeeds poorly, hand express or pump to relieve fullness.

- Avoid giving your baby water or formula supplements.

Sore nipples

Signs

Breast or nipple soreness can occur during or between breastfeedings. Nipples are pink, red, or purple. You may see a break in the skin at the base of your nipple or on the top of your nipple. Thick, yellow material draining from the damaged area can be a sign of infection.

Cause

Nipple soreness can occur any time, but it is most likely to occur during the first or second week of breastfeeding. Soreness usually occurs at the beginning of a feeding when your baby latches on to your breast and draws your nipple and areola into his mouth. If your baby is positioned well, the soreness will last only a few seconds. If your baby is positioned poorly, the soreness will continue and nipple damage can occur.

Other causes of nipple soreness include breast engorgement, breast infection, the use of creams or ointments, and the misuse of nipple shields or breast pumps.

Recommended treatment

- Position your baby correctly *at* and *on* your breast. Turn your baby on his side or tuck him under your arm so that his face, chest, and knees are facing your breast. Use pillows to support your baby at the level of your breast.

- Sit back or lie down, and relax. Bring your baby to you. Tickle his nose (or his lips) with your nipple until his mouth opens wide. Position your baby's lower lip against your breast and quickly but gently place your baby on your breast. His tongue should be over his lower gum, between his lower lip and the breast. His lips should turn out (not in) and lie flat against your breast. His chin should press firmly into your breast. His nose and cheeks may lightly touch your breast.

- If necessary, express a small amount of breast milk to soften your breast before you allow your baby to latch on.

- Begin each feeding on the breast that is the least sore. When a let-down reflex occurs and milk begins to flow, move your baby to the sore breast and breastfeed just long enough to relieve the fullness and soften the breast. If both breasts are sore, use a warm, wet washcloth and gentle massage to start the flow of milk before you offer your baby your breast.

- If necessary, limit the length of each feeding on the sore breast and breastfeed more often, every 1–2 hours. Hand express to relieve fullness.

- Hold your baby close to prevent unnecessary pulling on your breast. Remember to break the suction before removing your baby from your breast.

- After each feeding, put a small amount of breast milk on the nipple and areola of each breast.

- Wash your breasts and nipples once a day with a mild antibacterial soap and water. Don't wash your nipples before each breast-feeding. Even water, used often, will dry the skin.

- Avoid using creams, lotions, and oils. If your nipples crack or bleed, check with your doctor, lactation consultant, or nurse before putting anything on your nipples. Your health care provider may suggest that you put a small amount of modified lanolin, a glycerin gel pad, or a hydrogel dressing on the damaged area after each breastfeeding to ease soreness and aid healing.

- Modified lanolin is a purified form of lanolin. It contains less pesticide residue and free lanolin alcohol than other lanolin products.

Correct positioning

Incorrect positioning

Positioning your baby correctly *at* and *on* your breast will limit nipple soreness.

- Glycerin gel pads contain glycerin and water. Unlike other dressings, glycerine gel pads stay moist, but they absorb fluid. So when the gel pad gets thick and spongy, it's time for a new pad. Remove the pad before each feeding and reapply after.

- Hydrogel dressings are 96 percent water and come in solid sheets that can be cut to fit the size of the affected area. Hydrogel dressings dry out over time, so you will need to replace the dressing every 1–3 days or as needed. Remove the dressing before each feeding and reapply after.

- If pain, cracking, or bleeding occurs, you can continue to breastfeed, as long as your baby shows no signs of illness (e.g. vomiting, diarrhea, fever). If the cause of the bleeding is not easily seen or if the bleeding lasts for several days, contact your health care provider. While bleeding is seldom serious, continued bleeding can be a sign of breast cancer.

- If breastfeeding is too painful, you can stop breastfeeding for 24 hours and let the nipple(s) heal. During this time, you will need to hand express or pump to relieve fullness.

- If only one breast is painful, continue to breastfeed on the healthy breast. If both breasts are painful, feed your baby your expressed milk using a teaspoon, cup, or bottle.

- Thick, yellow material draining from the damaged area can be a sign of infection and may require an antibiotic. Contact your health care provider right away.

- A breast infection (mastitis) can occur when bacteria enter the breast through a break in the skin. Signs of infection include weakness, headache, nausea, soreness, chills, and fever (greater than 101°F or 38.4°C). If signs of mastitis occur, call your health care provider right away. A prescription medicine (antibiotic) may be needed.

To prevent sore nipples

- Position your baby correctly on your breast. If necessary, hand express or pump to soften your breasts and relieve fullness.

- Breastfeed as long as your baby wishes on the first breast before offering the second breast.

- Begin each feeding on the breast offered last.

- Breastfeed frequently during the day and at night. If you must delay or skip feedings, hand express or pump to relieve fullness.

- Use the breastfeeding positions that are most comfortable for you and your baby.

- Break the suction before removing your baby from your breast.

Blisters

Signs

A collection of clear or bloody fluid underneath the skin.

Cause

Blisters are caused by friction or pressure on the skin during breastfeeding. Blisters are usually filled with clear fluid but can be filled with blood. While the fluid can affect the taste of your milk, it will not hurt your baby. Because the fluid protects the new skin underneath, blisters should not be opened or drained. Leave them alone, and they will heal.

Recommended treatment

- To soften the blister and prevent cracking, put warm water on the blistered area before each breastfeeding, using a towel or washcloth.

- Position your baby correctly on your breast.

- Avoid breastfeeding positions that put pressure on the blistered area.

- If necessary, begin each feeding on the breast without the blister. When a let-down reflex occurs and breast milk begins to flow, switch to the breast with the blister.

- If necessary, limit the feeding time on the breast with the blister and breastfeed more often, every 1–2 hours.

To prevent blisters

- Position your baby correctly on your breast.

- Use two or three different breastfeeding positions each day.

- Hold your baby close to prevent unnecessary pulling on your breast.

- Offer both breasts at every feeding. Do not be concerned if your baby seems satisfied with one breast. If necessary, hand express or pump to relieve fullness in the second breast.

- Begin each feeding on the breast offered last.

Plugged duct

Signs

Signs of a plugged duct include a red, tender area or a small lump in the breast. The lump may or may not be painful.

Cause

Narrow tubes (ducts) carry milk from the alveoli to the nipple openings. When feedings are delayed or missed, or when your baby breastfeeds poorly, milk can collect in the ducts and form a thick plug or small lump.

Recommended treatment

- Put warm water on the plugged area before each breastfeeding.

- Breastfeed more often during the day.

- Begin each feeding on the breast with the plug.

- Adjust the position of your baby's mouth on your breast so that your baby's nose is pointing toward the plug.

- Gently massage the plugged area while your baby is feeding.

When feedings are delayed or missed, or when your baby breastfeeds poorly, milk can collect in the ducts and form a thick plug or small lump.

- Hand express or pump after each feeding to help remove the plug and relieve fullness.

- Choose a breastfeeding position that will best relieve fullness in the affected area.

- If a breast lump does not resolve within 2–3 days, call your health care provider.

To prevent plugged ducts

- Position your baby correctly on your breast.

- Use two or three different breastfeeding positions each day.

- Do not delay or skip feedings.

- If necessary, pump or hand express to relieve fullness.

- Avoid bras that are too tight or that bind, making it difficult to relieve fullness in all parts of your breast.

Mastitis (breast infection)

Signs

There are two types of mastitis, infectious and noninfectious. Symptoms usually appear quickly and include weakness, headache, nausea, soreness, chills, and fever (greater than 101°F or 38.4°C). A portion of your breast may be red, hot, and painful.

Cause

A breast infection is usually caused by bacteria that enter the breast through an opening in the nipple or a break in the skin. Factors that increase the risk of a breast infection include cracked nipples, plugged ducts, infrequent or irregular breastfeedings or breast pumpings, tight-fitting bras, illness, fatigue, and stress.

Recommended treatment

- Call your doctor. A prescription medicine (antibiotic) may be necessary. Although your symptoms may improve after 24–48 hours, take the medicine as directed until it is gone (usually 14 days).

- Put a warm pack on the infected area before each breastfeeding to aid let-down and relieve pain. Using warm washcloths or taking a warm shower or bath works well.

- Continue to breastfeed frequently on both breasts. The infection will not harm your baby. Breastfeed during the day and at night.

- Start each feeding on the uninfected breast until a let-down reflex occurs, then switch to the infected breast.

- Breastfeed only until breast fullness is relieved and your breast softens. If necessary, hand express or pump to soften your breast and relieve fullness.

- You can apply cold packs after each feeding to relieve pain and reduce swelling. Bags of frozen peas wrapped in a cold washcloth work well.

- Drink enough fluid to satisfy your thirst. Water and unsweetened fruit juices are best.

- If necessary, ask your health care provider to recommend a pain-relieving medication such as acetaminophen or ibuprofen.

- Get plenty of rest. Save time and energy by keeping your baby nearby.

To prevent mastitis

- Position your baby correctly on your breast.

- If you delay or miss a feeding or if your baby feeds poorly, hand express or pump to soften your breast and relieve fullness.

- Use two or three different breastfeeding positions each day. This will help to relieve fullness in all areas of your breasts.

- Do not delay or skip feedings.

- Avoid bras that are too tight or that bind, making it difficult to relieve fullness in all areas of your breasts.

- Wean gradually. Pump or hand express to relieve fullness and soften your breasts.

Fungal infection (candida infection, thrush)

Signs

Baby: Your baby can become infected during vaginal birth or while breastfeeding. Signs of infection often appear 2–4 weeks after birth and include small, white patches in the mouth (thrush) and/or a bright, red rash in the diaper area.

Mother: The mother can become infected while breastfeeding. Signs of infection include red or purple nipples, shiny areolas, and sharp, burning pain in the breast. Frequently the breasts look normal and severe pain is the only symptom. Some women also have a thick, white, vaginal discharge with redness, itching, and burning in the birth canal (*vagina*).

Partner: Candida can spread easily from one family member to another through close contact. Your partner can become infected during sex. Signs of infection include a red rash on or around the penis and small white patches in the mouth.

Cause

Candida is a yeast-like fungus that grows in dark, damp places. It can be found in the birth canal and on the nipples and breasts of the mother as well as in the mouth and diaper area of the baby.

Candida does not cause symptoms unless there is an overgrowth (too much).

Because candida is found in the birth canal of most women, babies can become infected with candida during vaginal birth. While the infection is seldom serious, it can be very painful. Sometimes an infected baby will refuse to breastfeed.

Recommended treatment

- Both you and your baby need to be treated, even if only one of you has symptoms. This will prevent reinfection. You may need to call your health care provider as well as your baby's. Your partner or any other family member (e.g., your baby's sibling) who has signs of infection should also be treated.

Use a clean cotton swab for each part of your baby's mouth (roof, cheeks, tongue, gums) when treating for thrush.

Mother: Rinse your breasts with clear water after every feeding. Your doctor can recommend an antifungal ointment such as Nystatin (mycostatin), Monistat (miconazole), Lotrimin (clotrimazole), or Bactroban (mupirocin). Put the ointment on the nipple and areola of both breasts after each breastfeeding for 14 days. If the pain is severe, your doctor can recommend a steroid ointment in addition to the antifungal ointment. Put a small amount of the steroid ointment on your nipples and areolas after each breastfeeding for 1–3 days; rub in well. It is not necessary to remove the ointment(s) before the next feeding.

- *Baby:* Your baby's doctor can prescribe medication in liquid form for your baby's mouth and in ointment form for your baby's bottom. Paint the liquid on the inside of your baby's mouth (cheeks, gums, tongue, and roof) after each breastfeeding, using a clean cotton swab for each part of the mouth. If you put a used cotton swab back into the medicine bottle, you can transfer the fungus from your baby's mouth to the bottle. If your baby's symptoms include a red rash in the diaper area, apply an antifungal ointment during each diaper change.

- Change breast pads and diapers frequently. Do not use pads with plastic liners.

- Boil all nipples and pacifiers daily for 20 minutes. Replace with new ones after the first and second weeks of treatment.

- Wash bras in hot, soapy water each day and rinse well. Boil all pump parts for 20 minutes each day.

- Wash your hands carefully before each breastfeeding and after each diaper change.

- Use condoms during sex. Do not let your partner's mouth come into contact with your breasts.

- If signs of infection remain after 5–7 days of treatment, you may need to use a different medicine. Your doctor can suggest another ointment or she may recommend a 1 percent water-based solution of Gentian Violet. Apply the solution to the nipple and areola of both breasts and to the inside of your baby's mouth (cheeks, gums, tongue, and roof) using clean cotton swabs. Use sparingly—a little bit goes a long way. The purple solution will stain the skin and clothing so be sure to wear a bra and T-shirt that can be thrown away. Apply the solution only once a day and for no more than 3 days.

- Gentian Violet can irritate your baby's mouth, so check with your baby's doctor before using Gentian Violet and discontinue its use right away if redness or sores appear.

- Resistant infections that do not respond to ointments or liquids can be treated with pills or tablets taken by mouth. Fluconazole (Diflucan) is approved by the Food and Drug Administration (FDA) for use in adults and infants. However, Diflucan should be used only if topical treatments (ointments and solutions) are ineffective.

- Discuss treatment options fully with your health care provider and your baby's. In addition, you may want to avoid foods that support the growth of fungus, such as alcohol, sugar, dairy products, wheat, nuts, peanut butter, dried fruits, and fruit juices.

To prevent fungal infections

- Wash your hands carefully before each breastfeeding and after each diaper change. Remove any artificial nails where fungus can grow.

- Change breast pads and diapers frequently. Do not use pads with plastic liners.

- Avoid using creams and lotions. They keep the skin moist but may encourage the growth of yeast-like fungus or bacteria.

- Keep your nipples uncovered as much as possible. You can open the flaps on your nursing bra or remove your bra for periods of time each day and at night.

Leaking

Signs

You may feel a tingling sensation just before your milk starts to drip or spray. Or you may simply notice a wet spot on your clothing.

Cause

Leaking is the result of the let-down or milk ejection reflex. When your baby breast-feeds, milk often drips or sprays from the other breast. Leaking can also occur between feedings.

Although leaking is common, it does not happen to all mothers. Leaking occurs more often during the early weeks when your baby's breastfeeding schedule is constantly changing. Once your baby has a somewhat regular feeding schedule (at about 6–12 weeks of age), your milk supply will vary less from day to day and you will experience less leaking.

Leaking can also occur when you think about your baby, when you hear your baby or another baby cry, when you delay or skip a feeding and your breasts overfill, or when you are making love and have an orgasm (sexual climax). Even a warm shower can cause a let-down reflex to occur and milk to leak.

Recommended treatment

- Use breast pads to provide short-term protection for your clothing. Breast pads come in all shapes and sizes. They can be disposable or reusable. You can even make your own pads using cloth diapers, cotton fabric, or men's handkerchiefs.

- Change breast pads frequently. Do not use pads with plastic liners.

- Choose clothing with light colors and small prints to help hide mishaps.

- Place a bath towel on top of the bed sheet. This will protect the mattress and keep the bed linens dry.

- Keep an extra nightgown handy just in case.

- Breastfeed your baby before making love or going to bed. This will limit the amount of milk in the breasts and allow time for sex or sleep, whichever comes first!

- Slow the leaking by pressing firmly against the nipple of each breast with the palm of your hand or your wrist, or fold your arms tightly across your chest. You may want to limit this practice in the early weeks since it can interfere with the let-down reflex and may decrease your milk supply.

To prevent leaking

Leaking lets you know that you are making milk. Leaking also helps to increase your confidence in your ability to breastfeed. If you try to prevent leaking, you may find that your milk supply stays low. So keep breast pads handy and allow your breasts to drip, drip, drip!

Chapter 15

Breastfeeding After a Cesarean Birth

Cesarean birth, often called a "C-section," is the surgical removal of the baby through an incision or opening made in the mother's abdomen. About 20–30 percent or more of all births are cesarean births.

Cesarean births are often unplanned. As a result, parents may experience many feelings including anger, relief, frustration, joy, and sadness. Discuss your feelings openly with your doctor, family, or friends. It may help to talk with other parents who have had an unplanned cesarean birth.

While a cesarean birth will not affect your ability to produce milk, pain and weakness may make it necessary for you to depend on others for help. If you or your baby needs special care, the start of breastfeeding may be delayed.

In the hospital

- Breastfeed as soon as possible after birth.

- If the start of breastfeeding is delayed for more than 24–48 hours, begin expressing your milk. The goal of early, frequent milk expression is to let your body know that a lot of milk will be needed in a few days. See Chapter 9, "Expressing and Storing Your Milk," for information on expressing milk. Hand expression combined with the use of a fully automatic electric pump with a double collection kit that lets you pump both breasts at the same time works best.

- Choose a comfortable position for breastfeeding. Use extra pillows to protect the incision and provide support.

- Position your baby correctly on the breast. You may need help with positioning, turning, and burping.

- Breastfeed whenever your baby seems fussy or hungry (at least eight times in each 24 hours). Breastfeed as long as she wishes on the first breast before offering the second breast.

- Increase the amount of protein (meat, fish, milk, eggs, tofu) and fiber (whole grains, raw vegetables) in your diet.

- Drink to satisfy your thirst. Warm liquids will get your bladder and bowel working again.

A fully automatic electric pump with a double collection kit lets you pump both breasts at the same time. (Example shown is Symphony by Medela.)

- Take short, frequent walks. Mild exercise increases bowel activity and helps you regain your strength.

- Get plenty of rest. If necessary, limit phone calls and visitors.

- Pain medicine may be necessary for several days. Your doctor can prescribe medicine that is safe for you and your baby.

At home

- Breastfeed whenever your baby seems fussy or hungry (at least eight times in each 24 hours). Some babies will not ask to eat often enough. During the first 2–4 weeks, if your baby does not wake often to breastfeed, you may need to watch for early signs of hunger or light sleep. Signs of hunger include sucking sounds, sucking movements, and squirming. Offer the breast when you see any of these signs.

- Keep your baby in the room with you to save time and energy.

- Get plenty of rest. Nap when your baby naps.

- Limit your activity. Avoid heavy lifting, household chores, and brisk exercise for 4–6 weeks.

- To promote healing and speed recovery, continue to:

  - eat a high-protein, high-fiber diet.

  - drink enough liquids to satisfy your thirst.

  - get mild to moderate exercise.

Use extra pillows to protect your incision.

Chapter 16

Breastfeeding a Premature Baby

The birth of a very tiny baby born weeks or months premature can be scary.

Why did this happen?

Was it something I did?

Was it something I didn't do?

Will he live?

Will she need special care?

How long will he be in the hospital?

Can I hold her?

How will he eat if he is too little to suck?

Can I breastfeed?

Premature babies can be breastfed even if they need special care. Breastfeeding gives parents a chance to share in the care of their baby, to do something that no one else can do, to parent in a very special way.

Even when you give birth prematurely, your milk contains just the right amount of nutrients to meet your baby's needs. In addition, human milk contains special cells that protect babies against infections, which are common in premature babies. Breast milk is easy to digest, which is important for premature babies with immature digestive systems. Also, research shows that premature babies who are fed human milk for at least the first month of life have a higher intelligence quo-

tient (IQ) at ages 7–8 years than babies fed infant formula.

Let your baby's doctor and nurses know as soon as possible that you plan to breastfeed. The hospital staff can give you information on milk production as well as the expression, collection, and storage of breast milk. In addition, they can put you in touch with other parents who have breastfed premature babies.

These parents, along with the medical team, can help you develop realistic goals and provide you with much-needed encouragement and support.

Breastfeeding even a healthy, full-term infant can be a challenge, and breastfeeding a premature baby can be overwhelming at times. If you get discouraged, you may find it helpful to know that premature babies benefit even more from human milk than full-term babies do.

As your baby's condition improves and your confidence in your ability to care for your baby grows, you will be glad you chose to breastfeed.

Feeding a baby who can't breastfeed yet

Your baby may be too small or too sick to breastfeed in the beginning and will need to be fed a special liquid through a small tube or needle that is placed in one of his veins (*intravenous* feeding). As his condition improves, he will be fed your milk through a small tube that is passed through his nose and into his stomach (*gavage* feeding).

Expressing your milk for your baby

- If your baby is unable to breastfeed, you should begin pumping as soon as possible after birth. Unless you are very sick, it is important to start pumping within 24–48 hours. The goal of early, frequent milk expression is to let your body know that a lot of milk will be needed soon.

- Ask your nurse for a fully automatic electric pump to use while you are in the hospital. Even if your baby is able to breastfeed, you may want to use a semi-automatic, battery-operated, or hand pump to increase your milk supply.

- Your expressed milk can be collected and fed to your baby or frozen and used later. If your baby needs to stay in the hospital for many days or weeks, you can rent or purchase a fully automatic electric pump to use when you go home.

- Each time you pump and before you handle the pump parts, wash your hands with soap and water and rinse well.

- Follow the directions for expressing with a breast pump in Chapter 9.

If your baby is too small or too sick to breastfeed, you can use a fully automatic electric pump while you are in the hospital. (Example shown is Elite by Ameda.)

- Pump *at least* eight times in each 24 hours. You will need to pump every 2–3 hours during the day and every 4–6 hours at night when awake. Many mothers pump every 2–3 hours during the day and sleep for 6 hours at night. Think of pumping as a special time to relax and picture what it will be like to hold and feed your baby. If you pump just before you go to bed, you will be able to sleep comfortably for a longer period of time.

- Many mothers get more milk with the first pumping session than with the next three or four, and then the amount slowly increases over the next several days. By the end of the first week, you should be getting at least 1 ounce from each breast during each pumping session. If necessary, talk with the lactation consultant or your health care provider about ways to increase your milk supply.

- During the first week, as your breasts change from making colostrum to making mature milk, they may feel very full. You will need to pump more to relieve the fullness and stay comfortable. This will help you build a good milk supply that can adjust to your baby's needs later as he grows. Though you may be making more milk than your baby needs, if you do not relieve the fullness and soften your breasts, you may never have the full supply of milk that your baby will need later. When the breasts stay full, your body will respond by making less milk.

- Plan to do some relaxation exercises at least once a day even if you cannot do them just before pumping.

- If you are able to pump in the hospital, sit next to your baby's crib, cot, or isolette; hold his hand if possible. If you are at home, make a phone call to the nursery to check on your baby's condition.

Storing your milk for your baby

Because freezing affects the anti-infective properties of breast milk, it is best to provide fresh, unfrozen milk each day if possible. Store your expressed milk in clean containers provided by the nursery. Glass or hard plastic containers with solid lids are recommended. Label each container with your baby's name, your name, the date, and the time the milk was collected. If you are taking any medicine, write the name of the medicine on the label.

Ask your baby's nurse how much he is being fed each 24 hours, and store your milk in 24-hour portions or single servings to prevent waste. If your baby is very small or not gaining weight, and you are pumping more than twice what he is being fed, pump the foremilk (milk obtained at the start of a pumping session) and freeze it for later use. Then pump the hindmilk (the milk obtained at the end of a pumping session) to take to the nursery.

The composition of stored human milk is affected by time and temperature. Recommended storage times are based on current research; however, research results vary. So, in the interest of safety, human milk intended for sick or premature babies should be refrigerated right away if possible.

When refrigeration is not readily available, human milk can be stored at room temperature (77°F or 25°C) for up to 4 hours. It can be stored in a refrigerator (40°F or 4°C) for up to 4 days, or in the freezer section of a refrigerator/freezer (0°F or -18°C) for up to 6 months (page 71).

Place all containers in the middle of the refrigerator or freezer section to prevent warming when the door is opened and closed. Storage has little effect on the protein and carbohydrate in human milk, but changes in the fat can give the milk a soapy taste, so always use the oldest milk first.

Getting to know your baby as his condition improves

As soon as your baby is stable and can be held for a period of time each day, ask his nurse if you can place him underneath your clothing and cuddle him skin-to-skin against your chest (kangaroo care). This early contact gives mothers and fathers a chance to care for their baby and to gain confidence in their ability to parent. Safe and secure against your chest, your baby receives all the warmth he needs as he gets to know you. Plan to hold him like this for about an hour at a time. The most stressful time for your baby is when he is being taken out of or put in the isolette, not the time he spends sleeping on your chest.

Both mothers and fathers can provide kangaroo care. Babies who are held skin-to-skin gain weight faster, move into an open crib sooner, and go home earlier. Also, mothers who provide kangaroo care often breastfeed for longer periods of time. You may notice that your breasts leak while you are holding your baby skin to skin and that you are able to pump more milk after providing kangaroo care.

Kangaroo care gives mothers and fathers a chance to care for their baby.

Beginning to breastfeed your baby

Talk with the medical staff about your baby's readiness to breastfeed. Recent studies suggest that a baby's ability to suck, swallow, and breathe in an organized manner is the best indication of readiness to breastfeed and may appear as soon as 32 weeks' gestation. Many babies can breastfeed, without showing signs of stress, days or weeks before they can bottle-feed.

Once your baby is ready to breastfeed, ask for (or bring from home) a pillow to support him at your breast. The football hold or cross-cradle hold usually works best in the beginning. Loosen your baby's blanket so his arms can hug your breast. Support his back, shoulders, and head in the palm of your hand. His ear, shoulder, and hip should be in a straight line so his jaw can relax to open. Express a few drops of breast milk onto your nipple and areola.

Support your breast with your other hand, and shape the areola and nipple into a wedge. Gently touch your baby's nose with your nipple. As he opens his mouth, continue holding your breast as you hug him to the breast. Resist the urge to press on his head, because that will make it difficult for him to swallow and breathe.

"Dancer hand" support is helpful for tiny babies with weak muscles. Using your thumb and first finger to form a U-shape, support your baby's chin on the breast with your hand.

If your milk is flowing freely, your baby may just lick and swallow. If your milk flows more slowly, he will start to suckle and swallow. He should suckle in bursts of at least six suckle/swallows (some babies do many more) and then will pause before suckling again.

As your baby slows down, you can massage or compress the breast to move more higher-calorie milk into his mouth. Remember that he has never had to eat before—milk was provided through a feeding tube—so he may not be really eager right away.

These first breastfeedings are a learning experience for both you and your baby, so relax and enjoy each moment. If you do not hear your baby swallow and your breast

"Dancer hand" support can be helpful for tiny babies with weak muscles.

does not soften, his nurse can give him your milk through a feeding tube (*gavage* feeding).

Often a mother is making more milk than her baby can take at first. If you are pumping 2–3 ounces per pumping session and your baby is being fed only 1 ounce per feeding, expect that he will soften only one breast. You will need to pump when you finish holding him. You may find that after your baby has breastfed you can pump more milk than usual for that time of day. Until your baby is fully breastfeeding, continue to pump after each feeding to soften your breasts.

If you are pumping more than twice what your baby is taking per feeding, pump one breast partially and then breastfeed on that breast. This will ensure that your baby is getting the higher-calorie milk, which will help him grow faster.

At first your baby may be able to breastfeed only once every 24 hours. The rest of his feedings will still be through a tube while he sleeps. Soon he will be ready for two breastfeedings a day, usually separated by at least one or two tube feedings.

When your baby is ready for a third breastfeeding each day, you will want to talk to the medical staff about doing two breastfeedings in a row to save you time and to see if your baby has the energy to feed at the breast twice in a row. As he gets closer to coming home, he may start to gag on the feeding tube, which is a sign that he is maturing. A feeding tube can be put through his nose and left there between feedings, or he can be fed with a cup or bottle.

Timing your baby's feedings

Premature babies go through several feeding patterns as they approach full term. If your baby is very small, he may start out with a continuous drip of milk into his stomach. Gradually a larger amount of milk is given every 3 hours—the same pattern as for a breastfeeding baby.

Then, often at about 34–35 weeks' gestation, babies seem to be able to eat more at one time, but they awaken less frequently.

If it is very difficult to wake your baby for feedings every 3 hours, talk with his doctor or nurse about moving him to a 4-hour schedule for a while. Expect that when he comes home he will change back to a 3-hour schedule as he gets closer to his due date. That is another sign that he is maturing. Since he is staying awake longer and getting more active, he needs to eat more often.

Providing a supplement/ substitute

Your milk supply may be low despite regular pumping, and breast milk (your frozen milk or banked donor milk) or formula supplements may be necessary.

If you follow each breastfeeding with a bottle-feeding, some babies can become confused. Milk flows faster from a bottle than from a breast, and bottle-feeding takes less effort than breastfeeding. So your baby

You can supplement your baby at the breast using a supplemental feeding device.
(Example shown is a Supplemental Nursing System by Medela.)

may learn to like bottle-feeding more than breastfeeding.

If you need to give your baby a supplement, you can use a supplemental feeding device while you are breastfeeding. A supplemental feeding device is a plastic container, filled with human milk or formula, which hangs on a cord around the mother's neck. A thin piece of plastic tubing stretches from the top of the container to the nipple of each breast, where the tubing is taped into place. When your baby breastfeeds, he receives milk from the breast and supplement from the container.

Once your baby is breastfeeding well and a good milk supply is established, the supplement can be discontinued. To ease your mind, you can weigh your baby before and after feedings using a special scale.

If breast milk production remains low, talk with a lactation consultant, doctor, or nurse about ways to increase your milk supply.

Chapter 17

Breastfeeding and Allergies

Breastfeeding a baby with a family history of allergic disease

The incidence of allergic disease has increased dramatically in recent years. The cause(s) for this increase are unclear. Genes play an important role in the development of allergic disease (along with environmental factors), which makes prevention of allergic disease difficult. But there are actions parents can take in an effort to improve their child's outcome.

Parents (expectant and new) who have a personal or family history of allergic disease such as asthma, hay fever, allergic rhinitis (runny nose), chronic ear infections, or eczema (itchy skin) should seriously consider breastfeeding their babies.

While breastfeeding will not prevent allergic disease in babies with a strong family history of allergy, exclusive breastfeeding for about the first 6 months, and continued breastfeeding for at least the first year, can delay the onset of symptoms (gas, diarrhea, vomiting, fussiness, and skin rashes) and reduce their severity. It's much easier to manage allergy symptoms in a 3 year old versus a 3 month old.

In the past, expectant and new mothers were told to restrict their diets in an effort to prevent allergic disease in their children. But recent studies suggest that exposing unborn and newborn babies to food proteins in the mother's diet (via the placenta or through breastfeeding) may actually trigger a more appropriate immune response rather than an allergic response. This theory lends support to the recommendation that mothers eat a wide variety of healthy foods during pregnancy and while breastfeeding.

It's much easier to manage allergy symptoms in a 3 year old versus a 3 month old.

CHAPTER 17

Preventing allergic symptoms

If breastfeeding is not possible and human milk is not available, your baby's health care provider can recommend a cow's milk– or soy-based formula. If your baby is extremely sensitive—or if severe symptoms such as vomiting or diarrhea occur—a special amino acid formula may be necessary.

Occasionally allergic symptoms develop in exclusively breastfed babies. Food proteins from the mother's diet appear in human milk in small quantities. For extremely sensitive babies, these proteins may occur in large enough amounts to cause allergic symptoms. In order to identify the cause of the symptoms, the mother's diet may need to be restricted.

Foods eaten by the mother that most often cause reactions in the baby are cow's milk, eggs, nuts, and wheat. You will need to eliminate these foods from your diet for 3 weeks, then reintroduce the foods one at a time, leaving 5–7 days between. It is unlikely that all the foods are the cause of the symptoms. By reintroducing the foods one at a time, your health care provider can determine which food or foods are the culprit.

If the restricted diet does not improve your baby's symptoms, you can return to a normal diet, but be sure to talk with your baby's health care provider about other treatment options. If your baby's symptoms are severe, a board-certified allergist should be consulted.

Introducing foods other than human milk

Parents have long been cautioned not to introduce solid foods too soon. However, some studies suggest that delaying the introduction of foods beyond 6 (or even 4) months, depending on the family history, may actually increase the risk for food allergy. When the immune system is exposed to foreign proteins (antigens) during a specific time period (not too early, not too late), a tolerance to the antigens, rather than a sensitivity, is more likely to develop.

Human milk is the only food your baby needs for about the first 6 months of life. When foods other than human milk are introduced, the new foods should be added one at a time at weekly intervals. This will let you clearly identify those foods that produce allergic symptoms.

Foods that are more likely to cause allergic symptoms are cow's milk, eggs, peanuts, tree nuts, soy, wheat, fish, and shellfish. Currently there is no evidence to show that avoiding these foods prevents sensitivity.

However, our understanding of allergic disease is constantly changing. So be sure to talk with your baby's health care provider before you introduce any foods other than human milk. This is particularly important if there is a strong family history of food allergy, especially peanut allergy.

Controlling everyday exposures that can increase the risk of allergy

There is evidence that early exposure to allergens, including infant-safe forms of peanut, may actually reduce a child's risk for allergic disease. However, if your child is already showing signs of allergic disease (e.g., runny nose, skin rash, chronic ear infections), the following suggestions complement the use of human milk in achieving the goal of fewer symptoms in allergic children.

- Reduce dust and dust mite exposure in the home. Cover your mattresses with special dust mite preventive covers, limit the use of wall-to-wall carpeting throughout the house, and change furnace filters frequently.

- Avoid bringing furry and feathered animals into the home during the first 5 years of a child's life. It is much easier to refuse a pet than to get rid of a pet that has become part of the family. If a pet is already in the home, early exposure to dogs, but not cats, may actually lower the risk of pet-related allergies. Talk with your doctor or your baby's doctor before you add or remove a pet.

- Keep infants and children in a smoke-free environment. This includes the homes of friends and relatives as well as automobiles. Early and chronic exposure to smoke is associated with an increased incidence of respiratory illnesses and early onset of asthma.

- Avoid child care settings, nursery school environments, and church nurseries. Heavy and early exposure to viral infections can cause chronic diseases such as ear infections and infectious asthma. Early and frequent viral diseases can cause a significant increase in allergic antibodies. If child care outside the home is necessary, choose a setting with fewer children to reduce the potential for problems.

- Breastfeeding, environmental controls, animal avoidance, smoke avoidance, and dietary management do not prevent allergic disease. However, in many cases, they will delay the onset of symptoms for many years and limit the severity of symptoms when they do occur. This will allow your baby to mature and be better able to handle any symptoms that do develop.

- Science has shown time and again that breastfed babies, both allergic and non-allergic, have fewer acute infections, less risk of chronic disease, and better response to immunizations. Human milk is truly the food of choice for every baby.

Chapter 18

Breastfeeding a Baby with Jaundice

Jaundice is a condition in which the eyes and skin appear yellow. Jaundice occurs when there is too much bilirubin in the blood.

During pregnancy, babies need extra red blood cells to meet their oxygen needs.

After birth, these red blood cells break down, and bilirubin is released into the blood. The liver filters the bilirubin from the blood and removes it from the body through the stools.

A baby's liver doesn't function fully until days or weeks after birth, so it is hard for even full-term babies to remove the large amount of bilirubin that collects after birth.

Meconium is a thick, black, tarry substance found in the lower bowel of newborns. Meconium contains on average 450 mg of bilirubin. Early passage of meconium keeps bilirubin from being reabsorbed into the blood and decreases your baby's risk of jaundice.

When rules or routines limit the frequency or the length of breastfeedings, babies have fewer stools, and their bilirubin level rises. High levels of bilirubin can destroy brain cells and cause lasting damage.

Jaundice occurs in 50–75 percent of full-term babies and 75 percent of premature babies. Because jaundice in the breastfed newborn is a common, complex, and poorly understood problem, treatment of the breastfed baby with jaundice often causes confusion and concern for parents.

In addition to making the eyes and skin look yellow, jaundice also causes many babies to be very sleepy and to breastfeed poorly.

Types of jaundice

Physiologic jaundice

Physiologic jaundice usually occurs 3 days after birth and disappears within 10–12 days. While many health care providers question the need to treat breastfed babies with physiologic jaundice, others recommend water or formula supplementation, phototherapy, or stopping breastfeeding for a brief time. Discuss the choices carefully with your baby's health care provider to avoid unnecessary confusion.

Phototherapy (light treatment) involves the use of a fluorescent or fiber optic light. When a baby is exposed to the light, her bilirubin level goes down. If an overhead light is used, a small mask may be placed over your baby's eyes. If your baby is placed on top of the light source, no mask is needed. Phototherapy will increase your baby's fluid needs, so remember to breastfeed frequently, at least eight times in each 24-hour period.

Babies with jaundice, especially those receiving phototherapy, may be sleepy, so you will need to work at waking them for feedings. See "Wake a sleepy baby," page 49.

Pathologic jaundice

Pathologic jaundice is caused by blood incompatibility or liver disease. Unlike physiologic jaundice, pathologic jaundice occurs within 24 hours after birth, and the bilirubin level often rises quickly. Prompt medical attention is necessary.

Breast milk jaundice

The cause of breast milk jaundice is unclear. There may be a substance in the milk of some women that makes it hard for their babies to remove bilirubin from the blood. Breast milk jaundice appears 5–7 days after birth. The bilirubin level usually peaks around 10–14 days and can stay high for several weeks or months.

If the bilirubin level continues to rise, your baby's health care provider may suggest that you substitute donor milk or infant formula for two or more breastfeedings for 1 or 2 days. Or, in rare cases, you may need to interrupt breastfeeding for 24 hours and pump or hand express. Because each of these options interferes with exclusive breastfeeding, discuss them fully with your baby's health care provider before you make a decision.

Breastfeeding jaundice

Breast milk jaundice should not be confused with breastfeeding jaundice. Breastfeeding jaundice occurs when babies are not breastfed often enough and appears 3–5 days after birth.

Breastfeed your baby whenever she shows signs of hunger (at least eight times in each 24-hour period). Fewer feedings result in fewer stools and increase the risk of jaundice.

Identifying the cause of jaundice

Sometimes it is easy to identify the cause of jaundice. Often a more thorough medical examination is necessary. Jaundice that occurs after your baby leaves the hospital should be reported to your baby's health care provider right away.

Preventing jaundice

- Breastfeed as soon as possible after birth. Colostrum is a natural laxative that makes your baby poop. Early, frequent stools help remove bilirubin from the body, decreasing the risk of jaundice.

- Breastfeed at least eight times in each 24-hour period. Frequent feedings result in frequent stools. After day 1, expect at least three stools a day for the next 4 weeks.

- Breastfeed well on the first breast before offering the second breast. This will produce high-calorie, high-fat feedings, which in turn will increase the number of stools and decrease your baby's risk of jaundice.

- Avoid using water or formula supplements. As long as you have a good supply of breast milk and your baby is breastfeeding at least eight times in each 24-hour period and passing at least three stools a day, your milk is all your baby needs.

Jaundice in the newborn.

TYPE AND FREQUENCY	SIGNS	STARTS
PHYSIOLOGIC JAUNDICE Affects 50–75 percent of newborns	• Yellow eyes and skin	3 days after birth
PATHOLOGIC JAUNDICE Very rare	• Yellow eyes and skin • Baby may be sleepy and feed poorly	Within 24 hours of birth

BREAST MILK JAUNDICE
Affects 1–2 percent of
breastfed newborns
	• Yellow eyes and skin
	• Baby is:
	  - alert and active
	  - breastfeeding at least eight times in each 24-hour period
	  - gaining weight appropriately
	  - having at least four stools a day
		5–7 days after birth

BREASTFEEDING JAUNDICE
Varies
	• Yellow eyes and skin
	• Baby is:
	  - sleepy
	  - breastfeeding fewer than eight times in each 24-hour period
	  - losing more than 7 percent of birth weight
	  - having fewer than four stools a day
		3–5 days after birth

LASTS	CAUSE	TREATMENT
Bilirubin is elevated for 10–12 days	• Breakdown of excess red blood cells • Immature newborn liver	• Breastfeed at least eight times in each 24-hour period • Check bilirubin level as needed
Bilirubin level rises quickly and continues to rise until medical treatment has begun	• Blood incompatibility (ABO, Rh) • Liver disease	• Medical evaluation • Breastfeed at least eight times in each 24-hour period • Phototherapy • Blood transfusion

Bilirubin level usually peaks 10–14 days after birth but can remain elevated for several weeks or several months	• Unknown; may be something in the mother's milk	• Breastfeed at least eight times in each 24-hour period
		• If bilirubin level continues to rise after 14 days:
		  - Start phototherapy
		  - Alternate breastfeeds and banked donor milk or formula feeds
		  - Interrupt breastfeeding for 24 hours

Bilirubin level will continue to rise until the baby is adequately fed	• Underfeeding—fewer than eight breastfeedings in each 24-hour period • Underfeeding—limiting the length of each feeding • Poor breast milk production, release, and/or transfer • Inadequate stooling	• Breastfeed at least eight times in each 24-hour period • Breastfeed as long as the baby wishes (baby-led feeding) • Confirm signs of milk production, milk release, and milk transfer • Supplement if necessary with breast milk or formula

Chapter 19

Breastfeeding More Than One Baby

You can produce enough milk to totally meet the nutritional needs of two (or more) babies. The amount of milk you make depends on the amount removed from your breasts through breastfeeding or milk expression. Early, frequent breastfeedings—or milk expression, if one or more babies need special care—will help you get off to the best possible start.

All the advantages of breastfeeding for mother and babies are multiplied when you give birth to two or more babies. Your babies benefit from the perfect blend of nutrients and anti-infective properties that breast milk provides. You benefit from the release of oxytocin that limits uterine bleeding, which can be greater after a multiple birth. You and your partner will appreciate the fact that breastfeeding requires little or no preparation and also offers cost savings. All will benefit from the enforced skin-to-skin contact that can help you get to know each baby as an individual.

Planning ahead

Be prepared to begin breastfeeding under many different circumstances. Surgical (cesarean) birth, preterm delivery, and other conditions resulting in a need for special care for one or more babies are more common with multiple births.

- Attend childbirth preparation and surgical birth classes early in pregnancy, beginning in your fourth or fifth month.

- Share and discuss information about breastfeeding multiples with your partner, family, and friends.

- Locate resources for buying or renting a breast pump should milk expression be necessary.

- Contact a breastfeeding support group or a support group for parents of multiples. Ask if someone can put you in touch with another mother who has successfully breastfed the same number of multiples as you will be having.

- Choose a health care provider who is knowledgeable about breastfeeding and who has cared for successfully breastfed multiples.

- Ask your partner, a family member, or a friend to stay with you at night while you are in the hospital, so that you will have extra help when you begin to breastfeed your babies.

- Arrange for daily or round-the-clock household help for several weeks after your babies come home from the hospital.

- Set a goal to continue breastfeeding for at least 6–8 weeks after birth, no matter how difficult it may seem at times.

The encouragement and support of those close to you, another breastfeeding mother of multiples, and your babies' health care provider will give you confidence in your ability to produce all the milk your babies need.

Beginning to breastfeed

Healthy, full-term multiples

Ideally, your babies' first breastfeeding will occur soon after birth. Healthy infants born at, or close to, full term usually search for and crawl to their mother's breast within an hour of birth. Although rooming-in, or a modified version of it, is possible with twins, you may need the help of a family member or friend if you have a surgical delivery or triplets. It is easier to breastfeed frequently when babies are accessible, and your confidence in handling them can grow when a nurse or a lactation consultant is available to help.

When rooming-in is not possible, ask that all babies be brought to you for all feedings. Each multiple is a single baby needing at least eight breastfeedings in a 24-hour period. In the beginning, it may seem confusing if each baby has a somewhat different, albeit normal, breastfeeding pattern. Until you have a better sense of each baby's breastfeeding style, it may help to write down feedings and wet and dirty diapers on a checklist that is color-coded for each multiple.

Preterm or sick multiples

When preterm or sick multiples need to stay in a neonatal intensive care unit (NICU),

you will want to begin expressing your milk within 24–48 hours of giving birth, if your condition permits. See Chapter 9, "Expressing and Storing Your Milk," for detailed information on expressing milk.

If you are sick and unable to express milk on your own, a nurse, lactation consultant, family member, or friend can help you use a breast pump. Do not worry about the quantity of milk you express. The goal of early, frequent milk expression is to let your body know that a lot of milk will be needed in a short time. The sooner and more often you express your milk, the sooner you will produce greater amounts of milk.

Most mothers find it easier to manage frequent milk expression if they use a fully automatic electric pump. When a double collection kit is used, it is possible to save time by pumping both breasts at once. Double-pumping also increases prolactin levels, which increases milk production.

Begin by pumping at least eight times a day. Pump at least eight times in each 24 hours for about 20–30 minutes each time. You will need to pump every 2–3 hours during the day and every 4–6 hours at night when awake. Many mothers pump every 2–3 hours during the day and sleep for 6 hours at night. To increase milk production for multiples, increase the number of pumping sessions as your babies' condition improves or any time you notice a decline in breast milk volume. Many mothers find that their milk production varies with the condition of their babies. By the time your babies begin to breastfeed, you will want to be pumping at least eight times in each 24 hours.

Sometimes one (or more) of your babies is able to room in with you. Or one is discharged earlier, while the other(s) must remain in the NICU. In this situation, breastfeed each baby who is with you at least eight times in 24 hours. You can pump for any multiple(s) in the NICU. To save time, pump one breast while one baby feeds on the other breast. If you don't think you are ready to coordinate pumping with feeding, pump both breasts immediately after a breastfeeding, or pump between breastfeedings.

Multiples with feeding difficulties

Multiples, including those born at or close to full term, are more likely to experience pregnancy, labor, and birth situations that can influence their initial ability to latch on and breastfeed correctly. One multiple may be affected more than the other(s). In addition, some preterm or sick multiples have difficulty making the transition to the breast because of exposure to other feeding methods that interfere with oral behaviors needed for effective breastfeeding. For example, the use of a bottle and an artificial nipple may interfere with the tongue placement and movement needed for breastfeeding.

These types of feeding difficulties may last from several hours to several weeks, but they tend to be short-lived. Most can be resolved with patience and persistence. However, "short-lived" may seem like forever when you are sleep-deprived and juggling

breastfeedings, supplemental feedings, and breast pumping sessions. Contact a breastfeeding mothers' support group and/or an International Board Certified Lactation Consultant (IBCLC) to help you. A support group or IBCLC can offer practical problem-solving strategies and provide moral support.

Developing a feeding routine

Almost any method of coordinating breastfeedings will work as long as each baby breastfeeds at least eight times in 24 hours. Some mothers breastfeed each baby on both breasts at every feeding. However, many mothers find it less confusing to feed one baby on only one breast at each feeding. This also makes it possible to breastfeed two babies at the same time. If you let each baby breastfeed as long as desired, so that your babies, not you, choose when to end a feeding, your milk supply will quickly increase to meet your babies' needs.

To stimulate milk production equally in both breasts, it is a good idea to alternate babies and breasts. You may alternate babies and breasts for each feeding, but many mothers find it is easier to alternate babies and breasts on a daily basis. For example, today Baby A (and Baby C) feeds on the right breast and Baby B (and Baby D) on the left. Then tomorrow Baby A (and Baby C) feeds on the left breast and Baby B (and Baby D) on the right.

Mothers of odd-numbered multiples may have to alternate babies and breasts more often than every 24 hours. If you feed the baby who wakes first, you probably will find that the one(s) feeding second on a breast, and last, will be the one(s) ready to eat first at the next feeding.

Some mothers assign babies a specific breast. Milk production in each breast then adapts to that individual baby's needs. However, you may find yourself with breasts of very different sizes! Also, you may find another multiple unwilling to breastfeed on the unfamiliar side if a situation arises in which one baby cannot breastfeed for a period of time, such as during a nursing strike (see "What are nursing strikes?" on page 60), which is more common with multiples than with single-birth infants. If you choose to have each baby always feed at a specific breast, vary feeding positions from feeding to feeding.

Breastfeeding simultaneously (two babies at once) can save a lot of time. Some mothers always breastfeed two; others never breastfeed simultaneously. Most mothers do both. They simultaneously feed two for some feedings and feed the babies separately for others. It usually depends on the babies' and mother's needs during any given feeding.

Don't begin simultaneous feedings until you feel comfortable positioning and helping a single baby latch on to the breast. At least one baby should be able to latch on and breastfeed without difficulty before you attempt to feed two at once. If both infants demonstrate any incorrect breastfeeding behaviors, simultaneous feedings may reinforce those behaviors.

Even if you or the babies find simultaneous feeding difficult to master in the early weeks, keep trying. It usually becomes much easier after several weeks or a few months when babies have become skilled at latching on to the breast. Use pillows to hold babies in position so that your hands are free to help with latch-on. Many mothers prefer the support of a firm breastfeeding pillow. You may want to work with pillows already available in your home before purchasing a special pillow, since some mothers find that pillows with a little "give" are more useful for positioning babies.

The following positions are the ones used most often for simultaneous breastfeedings.

Double-football/double-clutch hold

In this position, a baby's body is tucked under each of your arms (or is supported on a pillow at your side) while a baby's head is supported in each of your hands (or on a pillow). A mother's hands are free to help babies latch on when pillows are used to hold babies in place, so many mothers learn this position first. This position also limits pressure on the incision area after a surgical birth. However, it can be the least "hands-on" position, which is a disadvantage because it limits your ability to touch your babies.

Criss-cross/double-cradle hold

With a baby's head cradled in the bend of each arm and the babies' chests rolled to face your chest, criss-cross the babies' bodies in front of your abdomen. A pillow on your lap and under each elbow often adds comfort and support. You may be more comfortable if you place your feet on a stool, sit in a recliner, or tailor-sit (cross-legged) on the floor. This position increases skin-to-skin contact between mothers and babies and enhances baby-to-baby contact.

Some mothers adjust this position with older babies by cradling each baby's head and supporting a baby's body parallel to each of the mother's legs. To breastfeed in bed, a mother can lie on her back, and, with a baby's head cradled in each arm, lay a baby's body along each arm, parallel to each side of her abdomen. The babies' heads and bodies are rolled toward and face each breast.

Combination cradle-football/layered/ parallel holds

With Baby A held in the traditional cradle hold, Baby B's head is supported in your hand or on a pillow or "layered" gently on Baby A's abdomen. Tuck Baby B's body under your arm or lay his body on a pillow out to the side at a right angle from your body. This position lends itself better to discreet breastfeeding. It is a "hands-on" position, yet one or both hands can be free to help assist with latch-on.

Double-football/double-clutch hold

Criss-cross/double-cradle hold

Combination cradle-football/layered/parallel holds

Breastfeeding multiples simultaneously saves time and energy.

Partially breastfeeding

Full or nearly full breastfeeding is ideal for babies, but it may not always be possible with multiples. Partial breastfeeding provides babies with varying degrees of nutritional and infection fighting benefits. The benefits depend on the number of breastfeedings (or amount of breast milk) each receives. Regardless of the amount of breast milk provided, research indicates that any amount of breastfeeding, or breast milk, is much better than none.

Mothers choose partial breastfeeding for a variety of reasons. Sometimes they want some relief with feedings. Often partial breastfeeding is chosen because of ongoing feeding difficulties. Others choose partial breastfeeding when they return to work outside the home. Some mothers partially breastfeed, but their babies still receive only breast milk. These mothers pump their breasts once or twice a day, and their babies then receive the expressed milk from a bottle or cup.

Because breastfeeding means more than good nutrition to babies and mothers, fully breastfeeding one (or more) and fully bottle-feeding the other(s) should be avoided if at all possible. It may lead to long-lasting differences in a mother's feelings for her babies. In the rare instances when it is necessary, mothers should be aware of this concern and increase skin-to-skin contact with any bottle-fed baby.

Combining breastfeeding and bottle-feeding

Partial breastfeeding is more successful when bottles are offered on a limited basis. To maintain adequate milk production and avoid unanticipated weaning, breastfeed at least eight times each day. For example, breastfeed each twin at least four to six times in each 24 hours, each triplet at least three or four times, and each quadruplet at least two or three times. Remaining feedings can be expressed breast milk or infant formula if breast milk is not available.

Most mothers choose to offer a bottle during the night or in the evening when babies tend to cluster-feed. You can breastfeed first, then ask your partner to offer each baby a bottle to complement, or "top off," an evening feeding. Other options include your partner bottle-feeding one (or more) while you breastfeed the other(s), or your partner bottle-feeding all babies during one nighttime feeding while you breastfeed all during the next feeding.

Breast-milk-feeding

Mothers sometimes choose to exclusively bottle-feed expressed breast milk (*breast-milk-feed*) when one or more babies experience an ongoing difficulty at the breast. Short-term breast-milk-feeding can give a mother a chance to focus on increasing or maintaining milk production when pumping, breastfeedings, and supplemental feedings have become overwhelming. There are mothers who breast-milk-feed for longer periods. Some choose to continue pumping 8–12 times a day for many months and offer the expressed milk in a bottle or cup.

Returning to work

Employed mothers of multiples usually find it easier to continue breastfeeding when they rent or purchase a fully automatic electric pump with a double collection kit. Try to pump every 2–3 hours while away from your babies. If you want your babies to receive only your milk for their first 6 months, you may have to schedule one or two additional 10- to 15-minute pumping sessions each day to maintain adequate milk production.

Maintaining your perspective

Each of your multiple babies has the same needs as any single-birth infant, so multiples require more time and effort no matter how they are fed. Remembering this may help on those days when you feel as if you have competed in a breastfeeding marathon and have just "hit the wall." When you wonder if you will ever experience the "joys" of breastfeed-

ing, it can help to recall that your babies have been enjoying the benefits of breastfeeding and breast milk from day one.

Your multiples will be breastfeeding babies for only a brief period of time. Maintain your perspective by accepting all offers of help, surrounding yourself with a supportive network of family and friends, and finding the humor amid the chaos!

Confidence in your body's ability to make enough milk, and in your babies' ability to get all they need through breastfeeding, will grow as your babies grow. Before you know it, you will be numbering yourself among the many mothers who have successfully breastfed multiples.

Chapter 20

Breastfeeding an Adopted or Previously Weaned Baby

In a culture where many women have doubts about their ability to produce enough milk for their babies, it may seem impossible to consider:

• *relactation*—reestablishing a milk supply that has disappeared, or nearly so, or

• *induced lactation*—establishing a milk supply without a prior pregnancy.

Yet many women all over the world have been able to breastfeed their babies—both "homemade" and adopted—in these ways.

To understand how it is possible to relactate or induce lactation, you will want to refer back to Chapter 3. To relactate or induce lactation, you need the same three ingredients you need in the more usual breastfeeding situation: a breast, a baby, and a brain.

A baby's sucking stimulates the pituitary gland to release prolactin (the milk-producing hormone) and oxytocin (the hormone that releases milk). If this stimulation is repeated often enough, the alveoli (the milk-producing cells in the breast) will begin to do what they are designed to do—make milk.

Continued stimulation will cause the muscles surrounding the alveoli to contract and move any milk there through the milk ducts to the nipple openings so that it can be transferred to the baby.

It is as simple as that—in theory. In practice it is a bit more complicated. Because breastfeeding is a partnership between a mother and her baby, both of them need to be actively involved in the process. If a mother has little or no milk, her baby may be unwilling to breastfeed. And if a baby is being fed artificially, especially with a bottle, her interest in breastfeeding may be very low.

The mother attempting to relactate or induce lactation must find a way to do all of the following:

• Encourage her baby to latch on to the breast and suckle effectively.

• Ensure that her baby is being adequately nourished while she is building a milk supply.

• Maintain the special mother-child bond.

• Maintain her own interest and enthusiasm for breastfeeding.

Why relactate or induce lactation?

The usual benefits for both mother and child (physical, emotional, social, and economic) outlined on pages 6–7 apply when a mother relactates for her homemade baby. Many of the benefits also apply to adoptive breastfeeding, but because lactating in this situation takes special effort, it is helpful to review the benefits and ask which are especially important to you.

With both relactation and induced lactation, the long-term benefits are likely to outweigh the short-term benefits. In addition, the emotional benefits may be more apparent than the physical benefits—especially in the early days.

Some mothers need to wean sooner than they had planned. A mother and baby may be separated because of illness or other causes. Many mothers relactate because they want their babies to have the nutritional and immunological benefits of human milk. In some cases, mothers find after weaning that their babies can tolerate only their breast milk, and reestablishing a milk supply is a high priority.

Mothers establishing a milk supply for an adopted baby often do so because they know that breastfeeding promotes the development of the special bond between a mother and her child—a bond that would, with a homemade baby, already have begun during pregnancy.

Nutritional and immunological benefits tend to be dose-related. While even a small amount of breast milk is valuable, the baby who receives large amounts has more optimal nutrition and better long- and short-term protection against a variety of illnesses. Until a mother is producing significant quantities of milk, these benefits will probably not figure as prominently among her priorities.

Getting started

Getting started may be as simple as just putting your baby to the breast and seeing what happens. Young babies—and especially those who have had some experience at the breast—are more likely to be the ones who figure out what to do right away and suck at the breast as though they have been breastfeeding all their young lives. Don't assume that your baby is going to have difficulty just because she is a little older. Many older babies also take to the breast surprisingly well—even without prior experience.

Some babies may need a little help to latch on correctly (see pages 44–47); others may need encouragement to even try.

Helping your baby to take the breast

If your baby is having trouble latching on to the breast or seems reluctant to try, he will need a little extra encouragement. The following strategies have been helpful to other mothers.

- Keep your baby in close, skin-to-skin contact. Kangaroo care (see page 123) will help your baby get acquainted with you through his senses—smell, touch, taste, hearing, and sight—and, in addition, stimulates your body to release prolactin.

- Give your baby a chance to repeat the experience he had—or might have had—right after birth. Place him skin-to-skin on your abdomen just below your breasts. Stroke him and talk to him gently and let him explore at his own pace. Encourage him to seek your breast. As long as his inborn reflex to do so is still intact, there is a good chance that he will slowly make his way to your breast and latch on.

- Try taking a bath with your baby. Many babies who have difficulty latching on to the breast do better in a warm water bath. After one or two in-water attachments, your baby can usually practice his new skill on "dry land."

- Even during those times when your baby is not in skin-to-skin contact with you, keep him nearby so that you will notice the early signs of hunger, including:

  - squirming while asleep or awake

  - moving his head back and forth and wrinkling his brow

  - putting his hand to his mouth

  - making sucking motions and sounds

  - licking his lips and sticking out his tongue

  - making soft murmuring noises that grow louder

- Don't wait until your baby cries to offer your breast. He is more likely to show an interest in breastfeeding if he is in a light sleep, slightly drowsy, or just barely awake. You

can increase the likelihood of your baby learning to breastfeed by:

- keeping your baby near you during the day and at night. This will give your baby a chance to become familiar with your smell, to hear your heartbeat, and to find his way to your breast. In addition, sleeping near your baby at night makes it easy to take advantage of the increased nighttime production of prolactin.

- encouraging your baby to suck at your breast by using a nursing supplementer (see pages 125–126).

- gradually moving your baby from bottle to breast. A good first step might be to offer a bottle of your expressed breast milk or infant formula while your baby is held skin-to-skin in your arms. Some babies are more likely to attach to the breast if a bottle nipple or nipple shield is used on the breast at the beginning of the feeding. Over time you will want to remove the nipple shield and place your baby directly on your breast.

- keeping a positive attitude. Depending on your baby's age, experience with artificial nipples, and personality, it may take many tries before he readily accepts your breast. It may help to know that mothers who wean their babies from the breast to the bottle often meet resistance as well. They expect that it will take time before their baby warms up to a new way of feeding. Weaning from the bottle to the breast is no different. Your baby's cool reaction to your breast may seem like a personal rejection, but he is simply telling you that this new way of feeding is unfamiliar.

Feeding your baby a supplement

Whether you are relactating or inducing lactation, it is very common to have little or no milk when you start. Frequent suckling will stimulate milk production, but the quantity of milk produced may not be enough to satisfy your baby's need for food. Most mothers use infant formula to bridge this gap; others—especially those who are relactating because their babies cannot tolerate other foods—use donor human milk from a milk bank until their own milk supply is sufficient. Whatever you decide to use, it is important to make sure that your baby is adequately nourished during this period of rapid growth.

The nursing supplementer has the advantage of ensuring enough nutrition while, at the same time, ensuring that the breasts are stimulated sufficiently to promote good milk production. As your milk supply increases, your baby will take less food from the supplementer. Offering your breast without the supplementer several times each day will help your baby more easily make the transition away from the supplementer when the time comes.

Some families supplement their babies at the breast using a syringe, and others choose cup feeding and simply offer the breast for comfort during this period. If a baby is regularly fed by bottle, she may not suck effectively at the breast. But some parents do use the bottle for some of their baby's feedings. It is important to keep breastfeedings and bottle-feedings in proportion. Recognize the bottle as a risk factor that may make breastfeeding more difficult. But don't be too critical of yourself if you find that using the bottle sometimes makes this period a little easier.

Getting milk—when and how much?

The timing and amount of milk production vary quite a bit. It can be anywhere from a few days to several weeks before you see any milk. Once milk is present, you may go on to produce all that your baby needs—or only a part of it. Women relactating for their home-made babies are at a biological advantage. If you have had a recent pregnancy and produced milk for a period of time afterwards, you may find that your milk supply rebuilds more quickly and more abundantly than the milk supplies of mothers who have never been pregnant or were pregnant some time ago.

Your milk supply very much depends on the "baby" and "brain" parts of the breastfeeding equation. The baby's stimulation of the breast and the signals the breast sends to the brain are central to all breastfeeding situations. But emotions and beliefs also play a role.

If the mother is under a lot of stress, adrenalin and other stress hormones are released. Adrenalin works like prolactin to stimulate milk production, but, unlike oxytocin, adrenalin inhibits milk release. Stress hormones were useful in earlier, more dangerous times when women often had to flee with their babies. They were unable to breastfeed while on the run, but once they found shelter plenty of milk was available. Avoiding very stressful situations if possible, and learning how to relax through them if they are unavoidable, are adaptive behaviors that can help ensure that milk is always available.

What a woman believes about her ability to breastfeed is also very important. We don't completely understand why, but experience suggests that women who are confident in their ability to produce milk—and are supported by their families, their health care providers, and members of their community—often lactate more easily and produce more milk than women who are uncertain of their ability to feed their babies at the breast or have little support. This, in part, explains why breastfeeding tends to be easier with second and subsequent children.

To some extent, you can create a breastfeeding-friendly environment by selecting health care providers who support your efforts, by enlisting the support of family and

Creating a supportive environment will help make relactation or induced lactation a good experience for you and your family.

friends, and by involving yourself in a mother-to-mother breastfeeding support group such as La Leche League. You may not be able to eliminate all of your doubts about your ability to breastfeed, but creating a supportive environment will go a long way toward making relactation or induced lactation a good experience for you and your family.

Increasing your milk supply/ reducing the supplement

Once you start to produce even a small amount of milk, you will want to gradually reduce the amount of supplement you give to your baby. Keep in mind that every drop of mother's milk is nutritional and immunological gold, so your baby will benefit even if you have only a small amount.

Your baby will continue to need the supplement—at least at first—to ensure that both her body and her brain continue to grow well and that she has the energy to suck eagerly at your breast. If she is gaining nicely (5 or more ounces a week) and breastfeeding at least eight times in each 24 hours, you can steadily reduce the amount of supplement while maintaining or even increasing the amount of time she spends breastfeeding. Eliminating about 5–10 percent of your baby's formula intake at any one time is plenty.

Many mothers who find that they produce more milk early in the day (due to higher prolactin levels at night) prefer to reduce the supplement more during that period. They decrease three morning feedings by 1–2 ounces each, for instance. Some mothers are able to give a couple of breast-milk-only feedings early in the day or during the night and add the supplement to the other feedings.

There is no right or wrong way to combine breast milk and supplement feedings. What is most important is that you reduce the supplement slowly and check your baby's weight as well as the number of wet and dirty diapers frequently. No matter what your baby's primary source of food, you will want to see at least six heavy, wet diapers each day and one or more bowel movements, depending on your baby's age (see page 52).

If your baby goes through a sudden growth spurt, you may have to delay further cutbacks or even increase the supplement a little. This does not mean that you are producing less milk but only that your baby's needs have increased faster than your milk supply. With a little patience and careful attention to frequent sucking stimulation, you'll catch up and be able to eliminate more of the formula supplement.

This process may go quickly or it may take many weeks. Some mothers—especially those who are breastfeeding adopted babies—are able to eliminate the supplement entirely only after their babies are eating solid foods. For these mothers it is a long journey, but with the introduction of solid foods at about 6 months of age, their breastfeeding experience more and more resembles that of mothers whose babies were born to them.

Galactagogues

From the earliest times, many cultures have singled out foods and herbs that "make" milk. Such foods and herbs are referred to as *galactagogues*.

There is little evidence that these foods and herbs actually cause an increase in milk production, but the belief that they work may be enough to convince the brain (pituitary gland) to make more milk. Early relactation clinics in Africa often asked mothers to drink milk (an unusual practice for adults in that region), promising them that it would make their milk flow like the river Nile. This practice was just one part of a comprehensive program of support that enabled these women to resume full lactation for their babies.

Many breastfeeding mothers in Europe firmly believe that special breastfeeding teas are the key to a good milk supply. Most of the ingredients have not been proven to have this effect, though, and some of them—most notably peppermint—are known to decrease milk production. Only a very few commonly used galactagogues have been studied. All of them act on the pituitary gland to increase prolactin production and stimulate milk production. Among those that appear to be useful are:

- fenugreek—an herb previously used by dairy farmers to increase milk production in cows

- chlorpromazine—an antipsychotic drug

- metoclopramide—an antinausea drug

- domperidone—an antinausea drug

Research data with respect to relactation and/or induced lactation are limited. At this time, domperidone and metoclopramide appear to be the most effective, but caution is advised. Metoclopramide used for even brief periods of time can cause depression, and, although there are few known side effects with domperidone, the Food and Drug Administration (FDA) has issued a warning regarding the use of domperidone in breastfeeding mothers. Domperidone has been used with mothers of premature babies to help them maintain and increase their milk production over long periods until their babies are able to suckle effectively at the breast. It is best to talk with your health care provider before taking any medication.

Some adoptive mothers have participated in a program that involves the use of estrogen, progesterone, and domperidone given before the baby arrives, with continued use of domperidone afterwards. Initial reports from mothers are enthusiastic, although the amount of milk produced is similar to the amount reported by mothers who have had no medical intervention. And mothers with good community and medical support have also been shown to produce as much milk—with or without short-term use of either chlorpromazine or metoclopramide.

At this time there is no best way to ensure that a mother who chooses to relactate or induce lactation will have abundant milk. Women who live in cultures that believe that anyone with breasts can breastfeed seem to be at a psychological advantage with both relactation and induced lactation. But there are many exceptions to this rule. For the mother who wants to get her baby (back) to the breast and has enough support from the people who count in her life, it is certainly worth making the effort and seeing where it leads.

Deciding not to breastfeed

You may decide for many reasons not to continue your efforts to relactate or induce lactation. Perhaps your baby has been very unhappy with attempts to get him to the breast, maybe the effort involved has made it hard for you to enjoy your baby, or you may not have the kind of support you need to continue. In your disappointment, you may worry that you have failed or let your baby down.

Nothing could be further from the truth. By attempting to relactate or induce lactation—especially in a culture where breastfeeding is not the norm—you have already demonstrated your strong commitment to your baby's well-being, both physical and psychological. And because you are so aware of your baby's needs, you may clearly see that the delight you have in each other is taking second place to breastfeeding. Sometimes the best thing you can do for your relationship with your baby is to stop breast-feeding and shift your focus from producing milk to parenting.

If your baby is content to be at the breast, but there is little or no milk, you can continue to breastfeed him with a supplementer or switch to bottle-feeding and continue to use the breast to calm or comfort him.

If your baby is unhappy at the breast, bottle-feeding may be your best choice. You can still include many of the things you learned from breastfeeding.

- Always bottle-feed your baby in your arms so that feeding continues to be a social experience and a chance for you and your baby to be close.

- Watch for your baby's hunger cues just as you would if you were breastfeeding. Give formula on request so that your baby learns to recognize—and act on—his body's signals that he is hungry or full. Never pressure him to drink the last drop in the bottle.

- Use a nipple that makes your baby open his mouth wide. This promotes the development of his facial muscles.

- Choose a nipple with a small hole so that each feeding takes 20–30 minutes. If your baby still wants to suck after that, continue holding him and give him a pacifier.

- Switch sides to promote the development of your baby's hand-eye coordination.

This may take some practice because you, like most adults, probably have a favorite side.

- Your bottle-fed baby still needs skin-to-skin contact. Make sure he has a chance to touch you—on your face, your arms, even your breast—while he is feeding. Undress him a bit so you can stroke his arms and legs. A baby massage course might also be useful. Bathing together is another way of ensuring that your baby gets a sufficient dose of skin-to-skin contact each day.

- Keep your bottle-fed baby close to you by using a sling or carrier during the day and sharing a room with him at night. Studies have shown that babies who are cared for in this way cry much less.

- Talk with someone you trust about your disappointment and sadness that breast-feeding was not the experience you had hoped for. Letting out these feelings—and then letting them go—will benefit your relationship with your baby.

- Enjoy your baby, love him to pieces, and keep in mind that breastfeeding, however long it may last, is only one episode in the long story of your life together.

Chapter 21

Breastfeeding After Breast Surgery

Some women who have had breast surgery are able to breastfeed fully (without needing to give formula supplements) while others are not. Your ability to breastfeed will depend on the location of the surgical incision, the amount of breast tissue removed, and whether nerves, blood vessels, or milk ducts were damaged in the process. If the surgical incision was near the nipple and areola, damage is more likely to have occurred. As you think about your breast-feeding goals, it is important to remember that any amount of breastfeeding benefits you and your baby.

The most common surgical procedures are breast implant surgery (placement of breast implants), breast reduction surgery (removal of breast tissue), lumpectomy (removal of a breast lump), and mastectomy (removal of a breast).

Breast implant surgery

Breast implants are used to enlarge an existing breast or to form a new breast after one has been removed. Many women with breast implants breastfeed fully, although breast-feeding problems are more common in women with implants than in women without implants. Sometimes incisions are made around or near the areola for cosmetic reasons. These types of incisions are more likely to cause lasting damage to milk ducts, nerves, and blood vessels.

Since breastfeeding offers so many benefits, women with implants are encouraged to breastfeed. If you are concerned about the condition of your breast implants, talk with your doctor about a magnetic resonance imaging (MRI) exam. This exam can show whether breast implants are intact or leaking.

If you are planning to have breast implant surgery, let your doctor know beforehand that you would like to protect your ability to breastfeed as much as possible. Breast implants are usually filled with silicone gel or saline (salt water). Regardless of the type of breast implant used, complications often occur. Before you decide to have surgery, be aware that:

- Complications from breast implant surgery can include pain, infection, leakage, rupture, and capsular contraction.

- Breast implant surgery may affect your ability to breastfeed.

- Breast implants will make future breast examinations more difficult.

- Breast implants seldom last a lifetime. You will likely need more surgery to repair, replace, or remove the implants.

- Breast implant surgery and/or treatment of complications may not be covered by your health insurance.

Silicone implants

Silicone implants were first used in the early 1960s. More than 2 million women in the United States alone have received silicone implants. In 1992 silicone implants were taken off the market after several studies reported a possible link between silicone implants and autoimmune disease, a condition in which the body's immune system attacks the body itself. Since then, researchers have studied the effects of silicone implants on women and their breastfed children and have found no evidence of an increase in either breast cancer or autoimmune disease. Because of ongoing concerns about the safety of silicone implants, the Food and Drug Administration (FDA) determined that silicone implants should be used only in women participating in approved studies.

Saline implants

Saline implants are thought to be safe and effective and are approved by the FDA for use in all women.

Breast reduction surgery

If your breasts were very large, and you experienced physical or emotional pain due to their size, you may have chosen to have breast reduction surgery. When a large amount of breast tissue is removed, nipples and areolas are sometimes repositioned on the newly formed breasts. Milk ducts, nerves, and blood vessels are often damaged in the process. This damage can cause numbness in the breast and nipple which may or may not go away. This loss of feeling can affect your ability to breastfeed as well as your sexual response.

Women who have had breast reduction surgery often find that their milk production is limited. If you have had breast reduction surgery, you can still breastfeed, but you may need to supplement with donor human milk or infant formula if your baby gains too little weight. Let your baby's doctor know that you have had breast reduction surgery, and check your baby's weight frequently during the early months.

Lumpectomy

Removal of a breast lump seldom affects your ability to breastfeed unless the incision is on or near the nipple and areola. If a cancerous lump is found while you are breastfeeding, and radiation or chemotherapy is necessary, you may need to stop breastfeeding.

Mastectomy

Breast cancer occurs in women of all ages and is the most likely cause for breast removal. Breast cancer treatments include removal of the breast lump, removal of the entire breast, radiation therapy, and chemotherapy. If only a single breast is removed, you can breastfeed on the remaining breast.

Making a decision

Talk with your doctor (surgeon) before you have any breast surgery. Carefully discuss the benefits as well as the concerns. While your doctor will do his or her best to protect your ability to breastfeed, you may discover after surgery that you are unable to breastfeed fully.

As you adjust your breastfeeding goals, it may help to remember that any amount of breastfeeding benefits you and your baby. So make the most of your time together.

Any amount of breastfeeding benefits you and your baby. Make the most of your time together.

Index

About the author

Amy Spangler, MN, RN, IBCLC, is a wife, mother, nurse, lactation consultant, educator, and author. She earned her bachelor's degree in nursing from The Ohio State University and her master's degree in maternal and infant health from the University of Florida. Amy is a registered nurse, an International Board Certified Lactation Consultant, a former president of the International Lactation Consultant Association, and a former chair of the United States Breastfeeding Committee. Amy has worked with mothers, babies, and families for over 40 years. She and her husband live in Atlanta, Georgia. They have two sons, a daughter-in-law, and a grandson.

For more information about
our products, please contact:

baby gooroo
P.O. Box 501046
Atlanta, GA 31150-1046
Tel: (770) 913-9332
Fax: (770) 913-0822
Email: info@babygooroo.com
Website: babygooroo.com